Pocket Guide

to

NATURAL
HEALTH

BOOK YOUR PLACE ON OUR WEBSITE AND MAKE THE READING CONNECTION!

We've created a customized website just for our very special readers, where you can get the inside scoop on everything that's going on with Zebra, Pinnacle and Kensington books.

When you come online, you'll have the exciting opportunity to:

- View covers of upcoming books

- Read sample chapters

- Learn about our future publishing schedule (listed by publication month *and author*)

- Find out when your favorite authors will be visiting a city near you

- Search for and order backlist books from our online catalog

- Check out author bios and background information

- Send e-mail to your favorite authors

- Meet the Kensington staff online

- Join us in weekly chats with authors, readers and other guests

- Get writing guidelines

- AND MUCH MORE!

**Visit our website at
http://www.kensingtonbooks.com**

Pocket Guide
to

NATURAL HEALTH

*The Essential A to Z Guide
for Your Family*

Stephen Langer, M.D.
and James F. Scheer

TWIN STREAMS
KENSINGTON PUBLISHING CORP.
http://www.kensingtonbooks.com

KENSINGTON BOOKS are published by

Kensington Publishing Corp.
850 Third Avenue
New York, NY 10022

All Kensington titles, imprints and distributed lines are available at special quantity discounts for bulk purchases for sales promotion, premiums, fund raising, educational or institutional use.

Special book excerpts or customized printings can also be created to fit specific needs. For details, write or phone the office of the Kensington Special Sales Manager: Kensington Publishing Corp., 850 Third Avenue, New York, NY, Attn. Special Sales Department. Phone: 1-800-221-2647.

Kensington and the K logo Reg. U.S. Pat. & TM Off.
Twin Streams and the TS logo are trademarks of the Kensington Publishing Corp.

First Kensington Printing: January, 2001
10 9 8 7 6 5 4 3 2 1

Printed in the United States of America

To my beloved
Spring blossoms
In the heart of winter.
No one wants
This dream to end.
                    S.E.L.

For Joan—
On the pathway of dreams to you
My feet never touch the ground!
                    With all my love,
                    Jim

Contents

Acknowledgments	x	Bedwetting	49
Preface	xi	Bell's Palsy	50
		Beriberi	53
Acne	1	Bronchitis	56
Allergies	3	Brown Spots (Aging	
Alzheimer's Disease	9	Spots, Liver Spots)	58
Anemia	13	Bruising	61
Angina Pectoris	17	Bruxism (Teeth Grinding)	63
Anorexia Nervosa and		Burns	64
Bulimia	19	Bursitis	68
Appendicitis	22	Cancer	71
Arrhythmias (Irregular		Candida Albicans (Yeast)	
Heartbeats)	23	Overgrowth	77
Arthritis	26	Canker Sores	81
Asthma	31	Cardiomyopathy	83
Attention Deficit		Carpal Tunnel Syndrome	86
Disorder/Hyperactivity		Cataracts	88
(ADD)	35	Cavities	91
Autism	38	Celiac Disease	93
Back Pain	41	Cellulite	96
Bad Breath (Halitosis)	44	Circulatory Disorders	98
Bedsores	46	Colds and Flu	102

Congestive Heart Failure 106
Constipation 108
Cramps 110
Cystic Fibrosis 113
Cystitis (Bladder and
   Urinary Tract Infec-
   tions) 116
Dandruff 118
Depression 121
Diabetes 124
Diarrhea 127
Diverticulitis 128
Dizziness 131
Dry Eyes (Sjögren's
   Syndrome) 133
Ear Infections 135
Edema (Water
   Retention) 138
Emphysema 140
Fatigue (Including
   Chronic Fatigue
   Syndrome) 143
Fibromyalgia 148
Food Poisoning 151
Foot Problems 154
Frostbite 158
Gallstones 160
Gas (Intestinal) 163
Gingivitis 165
Glaucoma 168
Gout 170
Headaches and
   Migraines 173
Hearing Loss 176

Heart Attack 179
Heartburn and Hiatal
   Hernia 182
Hemorrhoids (Piles) 184
Hepatitis 187
Hiccups 190
High Blood Pressure
   (Hypertension) 192
High Cholesterol 196
Hives 198
Hyperthyroidism 200
Hypoglycemia (Low
   Blood Sugar) 203
Hypothyroidism (Low
   Thyroid Function) 206
Impotence 210
Incontinence (Involuntary
   Urinating) 213
Infertility/Sterility
   (Male) 216
Insect Bites 218
Insomnia (Sleepless-
   ness) 221
Intermittent Claudication
   (Poor Circulation in
   Legs) 224
Irritable Bowel Syndrome
   (Spastic Colon) 226
Kidney Stones 229
Lead Poisoning 232
Lupus 235
Lyme Disease 238
Macular Degeneration 241
Memory Loss 244

Menopause 247

Mercury Toxicity (Fillings and Environmental Exposure) 251

Milk Intolerance 253

Miscarriage 255

Mitral Valve Prolapse 257

Motion Sickness and Morning Sickness 259

Night Blindness 262

Nosebleeds 264

Osteomalacia (Bone Softening) 266

Osteoporosis 268

Overweight 272

Pellagra 275

Premenstrual Syndrome (PMS) 277

Prostate Enlargement 280

Pruritus Ani (Anal Itching) 282

Raynaud's Disease 285

Restless Leg Syndrome 288

Rosacea (Patches of Red Skin) 290

Scurvy 293

Shingles (Herpes Zoster) 295

Sinusitis 298

Spina Bifida 301

Stress 304

Stretch Marks 307

Stroke 310

Sunburn 313

Tinnitus (Ringing in the Ears) 315

Ulcers 319

Uterine Fibroids 322

Varicose Veins 324

Vitiligo (White Spots or Patches) 327

Warts 329

Wrinkles 332

Resource Guide 336

Index 375

Acknowledgments

A special salute goes to Lee Heiman for his home run in conceiving the idea for this book, for suggesting how it should be written, and for supplying some of the information for it.

We thank Joan Davidson-Scheer for sharing her wisdom in how the book should be developed, for her web research and verification of facts, her in-house editing, and computer reformatting.

We owe a debt of gratitude to the thousands of researchers we met only through their studies on which we based much of this book. They are the pioneers who guide us all to nutrients that make us more energetic, healthier, and wiser.

Just as teachers learn from their students, I, Stephen Langer, learn from my patients. Their teachings and experiences in preventing and overcoming illnesses are threads that make up the fabric of this book.

Our editors at Kensington Books—Claire Gerus and Richard Ember—deserve thanks for their multitude of suggestions for making this book more complete, better organized and helpful.

Many, many thanks to you, the reader, for your vote of confidence in selecting this book. We are grateful to you for taking time from your busy life to devote to the *Pocket Guide to Natural Health*. We hope that our book will profit you abundantly. May you be wealthy in health and healthy in wealth!

Stephen Langer, M.D.
James F. Scheer

Preface

The *Pocket Guide to Natural Health* is your "prescription" for preventing and coping with 119 common ailments. However, it differs from a doctor's prescription in an important way—it's readable! Further, you won't need a machete to hack through a jungle of unpronounceable, unspellable, un-understandable medical and biochemical jargon. English is spoken here.

We selected the ailments covered here from those that patients most frequently bring into the doctor's office—many that are not included in other books. We present research that has come from all parts of the world, not just the United States, because no single nation has a monopoly on quality health and nutrition investigation. Over and above this, we haven't omitted great studies just because they have a lot of miles on their odometer. Many of them are still invaluable cutting-edge research.

Likewise, we've included helpful data based on my findings as a specialist in antiaging medicine. Relative to clinical studies—usually similar findings by several doctors—we are more concerned with whether a therapy is nontoxic, noninvasive, and effective, rather than whether or not it's backed by an extensive double-blind study.

Even though most of our information is based on double-blind studies, all double-blind studies are not created equal. Some are poorly structured or draw the wrong conclusions from the right statistics. For us to print findings just because they are backed by double-blind studies would be like letting the double-blind lead the blind.

Usually books in the category of the *Pocket Guide to Natural Health* are published in hardcover or large trade paperback versions and come with price tags that are stratospheric. Our book is different. It was written to be a low-cost, original softcover edition that everybody can afford and also afford to give as a gift of health and well-being for family members, relatives, and friends.

We wrote this book in an accessible format and a convenient size that will fit in your purse or briefcase and become your constant companion. It will give you valuable health information in short "doses" that you can quickly and easily put to use.

One of the decisions we made while writing the *Pocket Guide to Natural Health* was not to include long lists of supplements that might require your having to mortgage the ranch to pay for them all! So we made careful evaluations and critical decisions, narrowing down long lists of supplements to those that will help you the most and debit your credit card the least.

This is *your* pocket guide to becoming and staying well. Take it with you everywhere you go for answers to all your health questions whenever they arise.

Here's to your health!

Stephen Langer, M.D.
James F. Scheer

Acne

Acne is double trouble—affecting both a person's physical appearance as well as his or her emotional well-being. Medically termed *acne vulgaris*, this disfiguring ailment results from inflammation of the skin's sebaceous glands. Glands become plugged with sebum, a greasy substance that they secrete. Acne is a disorder that is treated best in two ways: on the inside and on the outside. I see many patients totally healed of acne by combining the right dietary and lifestyle modifications with good habits of personal hygiene.

Recognizing Acne

Acne is characterized by pits, red scars, and pustules on the most visible parts of the skin: the face, neck, and sometimes the back and chest. It is most common during puberty, but can occur at any age.

What Are the Causes of Acne?

- Inadequate intake of water
- Diet high in processed foods
- Poor digestion (often due to a lack of hydrochloric acid in the stomach)
- Food allergies (especially dairy products)
- Nutritional deficiencies (especially zinc and vitamins A, B-complex, and C)
- Lack of exercise
- Stress
- Excessive cosmetic use
- Frequent touching of infected areas with unclean hands

What You Can Take

Nutrients

Name	Dosage	Benefits
Vitamin A	10,000 IU daily	Promotes healthy skin. Especially useful when combined with zinc.
Vitamin B-complex	100 mg daily	Needed for breaking down carbohydrates and fats to release energy. Cell energy contributes to healing acne.
Vitamin C	500 mg three times daily	Well-established ability to heal infections and wounds.
Vitamin E	400–800 IU daily	A powerful all-purpose antioxidant.
Zinc	30 mg daily	Healing teammate of Vitamin A.

Herbs

Name	Dosage	Benefits
Burdock	1 g capsule three times daily	Blood purifier that helps heal skin infections and irregularities.

What You Can Do

- ✓ Drink at least 8–10 glasses of pure spring water daily.
- ✓ Exercise regularly.
- ✓ Wash infected areas with mild soap to enhance healing.
- ✓ Avoid squeezing pustules as this can result in permanent disfigurement.
- ✓ Limit use of cosmetics.
- ✓ Relieve stress (*see* STRESS).
- ✓ Test for food allergies (*see* ALLERGIES).
- ✓ Avoid processed foods such as soft drinks, hot dogs, canned foods, heavily sugared breakfast cereals, and macaroni.
- ✓ Eat foods high in vitamin A, including eggs, milk, cheese, cream, butter, yogurt, salmon, bass, halibut, mackerel, herring, whitefish, sardines, tuna, clams, shrimp, beef, chicken, pistachios, pecans, walnuts, lentils, and soybeans.

✓ Eat foods high in vitamin C, including rose hips, acerola cherries, guavas, black currants, red peppers, oranges, grapefruit and other citrus fruits, cabbage, papayas, cantaloupe, and tomatoes.

✓ Eat foods high in vitamin E, including sunflower seeds, whole wheat, peanuts, cashews, almonds, walnuts, corn oil, soy oil, soy lecithin, spinach, asparagus, broccoli, oats, and avocados.

✓ Eat foods high in zinc, including seafood, sardines, oysters, soybeans, soy lecithin, kelp, legumes, meats, liver, eggs, brewer's yeast, mushrooms, poultry, whole grains, and pumpkin and sunflower seeds.

And Try This!

Try applying tea tree oil to affected areas every day, preferably after breakfast. It works like the conventional treatment for acne, benzoyl peroxide, but without the side effects.

Did You Know?

Lack of hydrochloric acid secreted by stomach cells is not usually a problem for young acne patients, but it is for 30- and 40-year-olds. I generally start the latter group with a combination capsule before meals—648 milligrams of betaine hydrochloride and 120 milligrams of pepsin—a standard formula.

Allergies

More than a generation ago, a brilliant researcher with a large practice, Dr. John W. Tintera, discovered through exhaustive review of the medical literature and his own studies a critical fact that seemed to escape others: weak adrenal glands prevent the immune system from dealing properly with allergens. Tintera often said, "There aren't different kinds of allergies, only one kind of adrenal gland—impaired." An allergy itself is simply an adverse immune response to a substance that is generally harmless. So while Tintera's position may seem extreme to some experts in the field, he was clearly on to something.

Recognizing Allergies

People often don't realize they are suffering an allergy attack because symptoms are much like those for a wide range of other medical conditions. Common examples include the following:

- Sneezing
- Watering eyes
- Clogged nasal passages
- Depression
- Frequent urination
- Itching
- Stomach distress
- Diarrhea
- Gas
- Fatigue
- Trouble concentrating
- Poor memory
- Arthritic pain
- Anxiety
- Bloating
- Blurred vision
- Cramps
- Dermatitis
- Earache
- Faintness
- Fluid retention
- Headaches
- Hives
- Hyperactivity
- Insomnia
- Irritability
- Muscle pain

And before running to the nearest allergist in search of answers, you can try two effective do-it-yourself tests for identifying food sources of allergies: the Coca Test and the Rinkel Rotary Diversified Diet.

The *Coca Test,* developed by immunologist Dr. Arthur Coca, works this way: Inside your wrist, find the area where you feel your pulse. Count your pulse for 6 seconds and multiply this by 10 to obtain a resting pulse rate for a minute. Take your first reading before you get out of bed in the morning. Repeat the process just after breakfast. Check your pulse rate again 30 minutes after eating a suspected allergic food and again 60 minutes after. If the rise from a normal base is 20 or more beats, you are probably allergic to the food and should omit it from your diet.

Dr. Herbert Rinkel's Rotary Diversified Diet works like this: Eat just a single food at a meal and don't eat it again until four days later. Then, when you do, if you are allergic to it, you'll experience a definite flare-up of symptoms. If you aren't allergic, you will have no symptoms. Repeat this procedure until you have tested all suspected foods.

What Are the Causes of Allergies?

Although allergy symptoms are numerous, their causes stem from just two main sources: food and environmental factors.

Allergy-provoking foods and food additives include the following: dairy products, wheat, beef, chocolate, corn, citrus fruits, eggs, coffee, malt, nuts, peanuts, pork, potatoes, soybeans, spices, tomatoes, yeast, wine, beer, dried apricots, oysters, salads from salad bars, all processed (packaged) foods, monosodium glutamate (MSG), sodium benzoate, artificial colors, and sulfites.

Just as there is an endless list of foods that can trigger allergies, there are just as many environmental factors that can do the same. The most notorious include: dust mites, pet dander, pollen, tobacco smoke, molds, cosmetics, bee venom, perfumes, smog, and cleaning solvents.

What You Can Take

Nutrients

Name	Dosage	Benefits
Vitamin A	25,000 IU daily for two weeks *Warning:* Pregnant or pregnancy-eligible women should take no more than 10,000 IU daily.	Strengthens adrenal glands.
Vitamin B-complex	100 mg daily	Necessary for maintaining the biochemical balance of all B vitamins when supplementing with any single B vitamin individually.
Vitamin B$_{12}$	1 mcg muscle injections daily for two weeks	Clears up asthmatic symptoms associated with allergies.

(continued)

Name	Dosage	Benefits
Vitamin B$_{12}$ (cont'd)	*Warning:* Vitamin B$_{12}$ injections must be administered under the close supervision of a physician.	
Vitamin C	1,000 mg three times daily	Strengthens immune system and reduces blood histamine levels.
Adrenal cortex (raw, freeze-dried from bovine sources)	300 mg three times daily	Provides adrenal gland support to deal with allergies.
Hydrochloric acid	Formula consisting of 648 mg of betaine hydrochloride and 130 mg of pepsin	Deficiencies implicated in 80 percent of all allergies.
Methylsulfonylmethane (MSM)	6,000 mg daily for three weeks, then decrease to 3,000 mg daily as symptoms subside or disappear	Flushes out allergens from the body and provides relief from allergic asthma.
Pantethine	600–900 mg daily	Powerful supporter of the adrenal glands and helps fight stress.
Pregnenolone	30–60 mg daily	Enhances adrenal function.
Quercetin	500 mg twice daily	Blocks the release of histamine from cells. Also stops the production of substances involved in inflammations.

Herbs

Name	Dosage	Benefits
Nettle leaf capsule	450 mg three times daily	Relieves allergy symptoms, especially itchy eyes, sneezing, and stuffy nasal passages.

What You Can Do

✓ Have your doctor check your stomach's hydrochloric acid level.

✓ Be aware that the traditional allergy scratch test is only about 20 percent accurate.

✓ Use the Coca Test and Rinkel Rotary Diversified Diet to identify foods suspected of causing allergies.

✓ Watch out for the most allergic foods: dairy products, wheat, beef, chocolate, corn, citrus fruits, eggs, coffee, malt, nuts, peanuts, pork, potatoes, soybeans, spices, tomatoes, yeast, wine, beer, dried apricots, salad dressings, and carbonated drinks.

✓ Avoid shellfish, because they live near the shore where water is often polluted by sewage and industrial wastes.

✓ Eliminate processed foods, full of additives that can trigger allergies, especially monosodium glutamate (MSG), sulfites, and sodium benzoate. Check labels when buying these items.

✓ Drink at least 8–10 glasses of pure spring water daily.

✓ Follow a diet high in proteins, including fish, meat, and dairy products (if not allergic or intolerant to them).

✓ Once you are cleared for allergies, eat the following:
  • Plenty of fresh fruits and vegetables.
  • Foods high in vitamin A, including eggs, milk, cheese, cream, butter, yogurt, salmon, bass, halibut, mackerel, herring, whitefish, sardines, tuna, clams, shrimp, beef, chicken, pistachios, pecans, walnuts, lentils, and soybeans.
  • Foods high in B vitamins, including brewer's yeast, liver, royal jelly, bee pollen, almonds, wheat germ, eggs, cheese, millet, chicken, mushrooms, soybeans, sunflower seeds, lamb, peas, blackstrap molasses, cottage cheese, sesame seeds, lentils, whole rye, turkey, and broccoli.
  • Foods high in vitamin C, including rose hips, acerola cherries, guavas, black currants, red peppers, oranges, grapefruit and other citrus fruits, cabbage, papayas, cantaloupe, and tomatoes.

✓ Don't smoke.

✓ Avoid alcohol and caffeine.

✓ Avoid sugar and other refined carbohydrates.

✓ Get plenty of rest.

✓ Exercise daily.

✓ Wash bed sheets and pillowcases weekly at a temperature of 130° F to kill dust mites that live on sloughed-off dead cells.

✓ Eliminate carpets and use washable slip covers on furniture, as well as non-allergenic coverings on mattresses and pillows.

✓ Prevent allergy-provoking mold by turning on heat in damp rooms and leaving a low-power electric light burning in a damp closet.

✓ Use humidifiers to moisten air if you live in a dry area.

✓ Vacuum often to remove pet dander and fur.

✓ Remain indoors during smog alerts and days of high pollen counts.

✓ Keep filters of air purifiers clean and replace them often.

✓ Replace strong smelling, skin-irritating bathroom cleaners with ecologically acceptable cleaners sold by many health food stores.

✓ Equip much-used rooms with a negative ion generator to prevent allergy attacks.

✓ Consult with a physician concerning muscular injections of beef adrenal extract if your adrenal glands are weak.

And Try This!

Try to rotate your foods, not repeating the same ones for more than five days. Clinical ecologists have demonstrated that eating the same foods over and over again can actually create allergies to them.

Did You Know?

Clinical ecologist Dr. James Braly, Medical Director of Immuno Labs, Inc., of Fort Lauderdale, Florida, believes that 80 percent or more of patients with food allergies suffer from varying degrees of hydrochloric acid underproduction. This deficiency makes it impossible for the pancreas to secrete enough digestive enzymes, so food is only partially digested. At the same time, the chemicals at work perforate the small intestine's lining, and incompletely digested food invades the bloodstream. This condition, called "leaky gut syndrome," may also be caused by drinking alcohol frequently with meals. Partially digested food particles, identified by the immune system as enemy invaders or allergens, provoke an antibody reaction.

Alzheimer's Disease

People often joke about having Alzheimer's when they're victims of everyday forgetfulness, such as losing a set of keys or not being able to remember someone's name. The disease, however, is no laughing matter. It is estimated that upwards of 100,000 Americans die each year from Alzheimer's disease. This condition involves the brain cells dying off at a faster rate than normal, while neurotransmitters used by brain cells to communicate are produced at a slower rate. The results are devastating, as anyone whose ever cared for a person suffering from the condition can attest.

Recognizing Alzheimer's Disease

Alzheimer's is primarily a disease of progressive mental deterioration to the point of eventually rendering a patient completely incapacitated. While it can strike at any age, Alzheimer's is most widespread among the elderly, affecting as many as 10 percent of Americans past age 65, and half of those over the age of 85. Symptoms may include:

- Depression
- Poor concentration
- Memory loss
- Dramatic mood swings
- Impaired space and time perceptions
- Poor abstract thinking
- Difficulty communicating
- Loss of bladder and/or bowel control

What Are the Causes of Alzheimer's Disease?

No one knows for sure exactly what causes Alzheimer's disease. The most widely accepted theories take into account the following factors:

- High levels of aluminum in the brain
- High levels of mercury in the brain
- High levels of beta amyloid: a substance that kills off brain cells and destroys memory
- Nutritional deficiencies (especially zinc and vitamins A, B_{12}, and E)
- Weak immune function
- Food and environmental allergies
- Family history

What You Can Take

Nutrients

Name	Dosage	Benefits
Vitamin B-complex	100 mg daily	Necessary for maintaining the biochemical balance of all B vitamins when supplementing with any single B vitamin individually.
Vitamin B_{12}	1,000 mcg under the tongue	Important in preventing dementia, depression, slowness in thinking, confusion and memory loss—all common symptoms associated with Alzheimer's disease.
Vitamin E	400 IU daily	Carries oxygen to brain cells.
Choline	2 g of choline or 30 g of 100 percent phosphatidyl choline daily	Is converted to acetylcholine, a key neurotransmitter Phosphatidyl choline has proven helpful in restoring mental alertness.
DHEA	60–90 mg daily	Significantly improves memory.

Name	Dosage	Benefits
DHEA (cont'd)	*Warning:* Take only under the supervision of a physician. Do not take if you are at risk of hormone-related cancer.	
Zinc	50–100 mg daily	Prevents formation of amyloid plaque.

Herbs

Name	Dosage	Benefits
Ginkgo biloba	80 mg three times daily	Improves blood flow throughout the body. Delays decline of mental efficiency and improves memory.

What You Can Do

✓ Take a hair analysis test for toxic levels of heavy metals in the body.
✓ Test for food and environmental allergies (*see* ALLERGIES).
✓ Avoid alcohol.
✓ Test your water for alum, a variety of aluminum, used to settle impurities in municipal water supplies. Levels of alum differ in each community. At .03 or higher there may be danger to you and your loved ones.
✓ Avoid these foods: nondairy creamers, processed foods (read labels carefully), baking powder, biscuit dough, bleached white flour, some cheeses and cheese sauces, pickles (look for the label ingredient alum), some salad dressings, and salt.
✓ Check for hidden sources of aluminum, including: antacids, antidiarrhea formulas, antiperspirants, buffered aspirin, metal containers, cooking utensils, deodorants, douches, feminine hygiene formulas, certain hemorrhoid salves, lip rouge, some lotions, skin creams, and certain toothpastes.

✓ Consider replacing your mercury amalgam fillings. Studies have shown direct correlations between toxic mercury levels in the brain and the number of mercury fillings in the mouth.

✓ Eat foods high in vitamin B_{12}, including liver, sardines, mackerel, herring, red snapper, flounder, salmon, lamb, Swiss cheese, blue cheese, eggs, haddock, beef, halibut, anchovies, chicken, turkey, milk, and butter.

✓ Eat foods high in vitamin E, including sunflower seeds, whole wheat, peanuts, cashews, almonds, walnuts, corn oil, soy oil, soy lecithin, spinach, asparagus, broccoli, oats, and avocados.

✓ Eat foods high in choline, including whole grains, soybeans, soy lecithin, meat, milk, eggs, and legumes.

✓ Eat foods high in zinc, including seafood, sardines, oysters, soybeans, soy lecithin, kelp, legumes, meats, liver, eggs, brewer's yeast, mushrooms, poultry, whole grains, and pumpkin and sunflower seeds.

And Try This!

Try chelation therapy, a safe and effective means of ridding the body of heavy toxic metals such as aluminum and mercury. Chelation therapy can be performed either orally or intravenously and has been used successfully in the treatment of Alzheimer's disease. Please consult with a physician trained in this practice, as it requires close medical supervision.

Did You Know?

A 10-year British government survey of 4,000 adults, ages 49 to 69, in 88 counties of England and Wales compared the incidence of Alzheimer's disease and the amounts of aluminum in local water sources, revealing that individuals who drank water with the highest aluminum content had a 50 percent greater risk of developing Alzheimer's disease than those whose water contained no aluminum.

Anemia

The word *anemia* comes from the Greek, meaning "lacking blood." Anemia patients generally have enough blood, but not enough red blood cells or enough hemoglobin (red coloring) in the blood. This leads to a reduction of oxygen in additional cells throughout the body—a dangerous and potentially deadly condition. More than 100 different types of anemia have been identified, with the most common including pernicious anemia (vitamin B_{12} deficiency), folic acid deficiency anemia, and sickle cell anemia.

Recognizing Anemia

Half of all anemia cases occur in children. Anemia is also not easy to detect and often goes undiagnosed. While a major health problem in its own right, it can be a sign of even more serious illness as well. Symptoms of anemia may include:

- Fatigue
- Paleness (skin, lips, and nails)
- Appetite loss
- Red, swollen, and sore tongue
- Shortness of breath
- Diarrhea
- Constipation
- Headaches
- Confusion
- Disorientation
- Failing memory
- Depression
- Poor reflexes
- Prickling sensation or numbness in the legs
- Nervous system and heart disorders
- Lack of menstruation

What Are the Causes of Anemia?

Anything that interferes with the production of red blood cells or destroys them too quickly can cause anemia. Iron deficiency is the primary culprit, as it is central to the formation of red blood cells and of hemoglobin.

Specific types of anemia may be related to other factors just as important. *Pernicious anemia* results from a deficiency in vitamin B_{12}, and is often associated with a strict vegetarian diet.

Folic acid deficiency anemia occurs when this vitamin is lacking in the diet, mainly from a failure to eat enough fruits and vegetables or alcohol abuse. *Sickle cell anemia* is a hereditary condition where cells are literally shaped like a sickle, making oxygen release difficult.

Factors known to cause anemia include the following:

- Iron deficiency
- Vitamin B$_{12}$ deficiency
- Folic acid deficiency
- Zinc deficiency
- Family history (sickle cell anemia)
- Poor digestion (lack of hydrochloric acid in the stomach)
- Alcoholism
- Drug use
- Heavy menstruation
- Arthritis
- Liver damage
- Thyroid disorders
- Infections
- Multiple pregnancies

What You Can Take

Nutrients

Name	Dosage	Benefits
Iron	Consult with physician. *Warning:* Iron should only be taken under close medical supervision once anemia has been diagnosed since severe side effects may occur from improper dosage.	Deficiencies linked to anemia.
Folic acid	400 mcg tablet after each meal for folic acid-deficiency patients. 5 mg daily (megadose) daily for sickle cell only	Essential for red blood cell formation.
Vitamin B$_6$	50 mg twice daily. Sickle cell only	Enhances absorption of vitamin B$_{12}$.
Vitamin B$_{12}$	Ten 1,000 mcg pellets under the tongue daily in place of injections	Essential for red blood cell formation.

Name	Dosage	Benefits
Vitamin B$_{12}$ (cont'd)	then return to one 1,000 mcg pellet three times daily when the pernicious anemia is over (maintenance dosage)	
Vitamin B-complex	100 mg daily.	Necessary for maintaining the biochemical balance of all B vitamins when supplementing with any single B vitamin.
Vitamin E	450 IU daily	May reduce the number of irreversibly sickled cells. Helps prolong life of red blood cells.
Glutathione	100 mcg daily for sickle cell only	Protects red blood cells from free radical damage.
Selenium	200 mcg daily	Protects red blood cells from free radical damage.
Zinc	15 mg tablets six times daily	A must for sickle cell anemia patients. Prevents red blood cells from becoming deformed into the sickle shape.

What You Can Do

✓ Have blood checked if you are pale, energy-depleted, and low in spirits.
✓ Eat plenty of fresh fruits and vegetables daily (especially for folic acid anemia).
✓ Avoid alcohol.
✓ Eat liver, meat, poultry, fish, and eggs to prevent pernicious anemia.
✓ Be sure to take supplemental vitamin B$_{12}$ if you are vegetarian.
✓ Eat foods high in the following nutrients:
  • Iron, including brewer's yeast, soy lecithin, pumpkin and sesame seeds, wheat germ, blackstrap molasses, liver, eggs, millet, lentils, walnuts, almonds, raisins, and oats.

- Folic acid, including whole grains, wheat germ, bran, brown rice, liver, milk, beef, barley, chicken, tuna, salmon, lentils, legumes, brewer's yeast, cheese, oranges, mushrooms, and green leafy vegetables.
- Vitamin B_6, including brewer's yeast, brown rice, whole wheat, royal jelly, soybeans, rye, lentils, sunflower seeds, alfalfa, salmon, wheat germ, tuna, bran, walnuts, cashews, peanuts, peas, liver, avocados, beans, turkey, oats, chicken, halibut, lamb, and bananas.
- Vitamin B_{12}, including liver, sardines, mackerel, herring, red snapper, flounder, salmon, lamb, Swiss cheese, blue cheese, eggs, haddock, beef, halibut, anchovies, chicken, turkey, milk, and butter.
- Vitamin E, including sunflower seeds, whole wheat, peanuts, cashews, almonds, walnuts, corn oil, soy oil, soy lecithin, spinach, asparagus, broccoli, oats, and avocados.
- Selenium, including Brazil nuts, fish, organ meats, whole grains, eggs, cabbage, corn, peas, onions, garlic, chicken, beets, barley, and tomatoes.
- Zinc, including seafood, sardines, oysters, soybeans, soy lecithin, kelp, legumes, meats, liver, eggs, brewer's yeast, mushrooms, poultry, whole grains, and pumpkin and sunflower seeds.

And Try This!

Try taking a tablespoon of blackstrap molasses once in the morning and once at night. It's high in both iron and B vitamins—and it's a tasty snack!

Did You Know?

In 1926 Drs. George R. Minot and William P. Murphy discovered that intramuscular injections of raw liver extract could control pernicious anemia. This discovery saved countless lives and won the Nobel Prize in medicine. Other doctors had their patients eat several pounds of beef liver daily until they could no longer tolerate it. When researchers found that the curative factor in liver was vitamin B_{12}, they learned that

1 mcg (microgram) of vitamin B_{12} injected daily for a week reversed pernicious anemia—even today, this is still a standard treatment.

Angina Pectoris

Angina pectoris simply means "chest pain." In this case, the pain is due to a constriction or spasm of the coronary arteries—those that supply blood to the heart. A chest pain that occasionally radiates to the arms, the back, and even the jaw is the body's warning that the heart muscle desperately needs oxygen. This is sometimes mistaken for pain from indigestion. However, in most instances, the difference is marked.

Recognizing Angina Pectoris

"You feel as if an elephant is sitting on your chest and crushing it," an angina patient once told me. "The pain is excruciating!" He wasn't kidding. The chest pain may indeed be this severe but it may also be mild. In either case, it often accompanies or follows physical exertion and can be a forerunner to a heart attack.

Warning: Always contact your doctor or get to a hospital immediately upon experiencing severe chest pain.

What Are the Causes of Angina Pectoris?

- Diabetes
- Smoking
- High blood pressure
- Elevated levels of uric acid, fibrinogen (a clotting agent), or homocysteine, a chemical by-product of the metabolism of the amino acid methionine

What You Can Take

Nutrients

Name	Dosage	Benefits
Arginine	2–4 teaspoons daily, which is the equivalent of 8-16 g *Warning:* Do not take if you have kidney disease, genital herpes, or repeated cold sores.	Amino acid that reduces angina pain.
Beta-carotene	50 mg daily	Reduces angina pain, and promotes a healthy heart in general.
L-carnitine	3.5 g daily	Reduces angina pain.

What You Can Do

✓ Keep nitroglycerine capsules, pellets, or spray on hand for an emergency (as prescribed by your doctor).
✓ Speak to a physician trained in chelation therapy, a safe and effective means of ridding the body of heavy toxic metals such as aluminum and mercury. Chelation therapy can be performed either orally or intravenously and has been used successfully in the treatment of arterial blockage, which causes angina pectoris.

And Try This!

Try sipping from a cupful of tea made from hawthorn leaves three times daily, as it is an effective dilator of the arteries. Hawthorn must not be used, however, if you are taking digitalis medications.

Did You Know?

A research project reported in the *Medical Tribune* demonstrated that 333 patients on 50 mg (83,350 IU) every other day of the antioxidant beta-carotene reduced their heart ailments by about 50 percent, compared with those who didn't take this supplement. Angina patients particularly benefited, experiencing far less intense heart pains.

Anorexia Nervosa and Bulimia

Anorexia nervosa and bulimia are not the same illness but can be similar in both cause and effect. Treatment for each also often overlaps. Anorexia is best characterized as starving oneself to become thin. Bulimia also stems from an extreme phobia of gaining weight, but rather than refuse to eat, bulimics tend to stuff themselves with food (binge) and then "purge" by forcing themselves to vomit and take cathartics. An estimated one-third of high school and college-age young women suffer from these eating disorders.

Recognizing Anorexia Nervosa and Bulimia

No matter what cover-ups they use to hide their conduct, anorexics and bulimics eventually reveal themselves. Warning signs may include:

- Rushing to the bathroom to throw up during or after meals
- Sour breath from the smell of stomach acids
- Sore throat from vomiting
- Runny nose from vomiting
- Tooth enamel that is stained brown or etched from stomach acids
- Irregular menstrual cycle (it often stops)
- Laxative abuse
- Excessive exercising
- Underweight
- Obsession with food
- Ritualized eating patterns (e.g. cutting things into tiny portions)
- General physical weakness

- Broken blood vessels in the face
- Low blood pressure
- Dizziness
- Depression
- Mood swings
- Thyroid dysfunction
- Irregular heartbeats
- Muscle spasms
- Dehydration

What Are the Causes of Anorexia Nervosa and Bulimia?

Anorexia and bulimia are considered to be primarily psychological disorders—at least in origin. Apart from the obvious social influences screaming at women to be supermodel-thin, some psychotherapists believe there's more to the problem than a desire to look gaunt. Starvation can be a young girl's subconscious way of refusing to enter puberty. Her rejection of developing breasts, menstruation, and other signs of maturing demonstrate her desire to remain in a state of childish dependency. Other experts in the field cite additional factors:

- Low self-esteem
- Depression
- Perfectionism
- Feeling unloved
- Loneliness
- Peer pressure
- Inferiority complex
- Chemical imbalances
- Lack of zinc (can suppress appetite)

What You Can Take

Nutrients

Name	Dosage	Benefits
Vitamin B-complex	100 mg daily	Increases energy and stimulates appetite.
Zinc	30 mg daily	Excellent for stimulating appetite.
Multivitamin and mineral complex	As directed on label	All nutrients are needed, as condition leads to general deficiencies.

What You Can Do

✓ Both psychological and physiological aspects of this illness must be treated. The best way to begin is by seeing a trained counselor who specializes in the unique psychological aspects of eating disorders.

✓ In addition to seeking professional help, I suggest starting out with a light diet of vegetables and fruit with a small amount of protein (to be increased steadily).

✓ Eat foods high in zinc, including almonds, avocados, beef, bleu cheese, blackstrap molasses, brewer's yeast, buckwheat, chicken, cocoa, corn, egg yolk, lamb, liver, millet, oats, peas, rye, soybeans, sunflower seeds, turkey, walnuts, wheat, and whole-grain rice.

And Try This!

Try a tablespoon of royal jelly twice daily either straight from the spoon or on toast or cereal. Royal jelly contains all eight essential amino acids, all the B vitamins, and the minerals calcium, copper, iron, phosphorus, potassium, silica, and sulfur. It's been used by English royals to cure anorexia. And of course, queen bees swear by it. Not to mention the fact that it tastes great!

Did You Know?

In a study by biochemists R. L. Casper and J. M. Davis, published in the *American Journal of Clinical Nutrition,* 30 hospitalized anorexics were found to be zinc-deficient. They could hardly distinguish the difference between sour and bitter foods. Along with food, they were given 30 mg of zinc daily. Within less than a week, their ability to taste foods improved. So did their appetites.

Appendicitis

Your appendix is a 2- to 6-inch tube that looks like a thick worm, with an opening next to the upward part of the large intestine and blockage at the other end. There's always a danger, when a person is constipated, that pellets of waste matter will back up and enter the appendix and putrefy there. Bacterial action makes this waste matter more toxic, causing inflammation and gas that create pain—especially in the lower right abdomen away from the belly button—nausea, and possible vomiting. The appendix swells even more, threatening to burst. If it does (appendicitis), there's an explosion of poisons throughout the system. The victim then is closer to dying than living—unless the emergency room personnel can work wonders.

Recognizing Appendicitis

- Painful gas (often excruciating) in the lower right abdomen
- Acute pain in the lower right abdomen when pressed
- Abdominal pain that may become worse when walking or coughing
- Fever
- Loss of appetite
- Nausea
- Possible vomiting

Warning: Get to a hospital immediately at the first sign of appendicitis.

What Is the Cause of Appendicitis?

- Infection from intestinal bacteria

What You Can Do

✓ Avoid constipation (*see* CONSTIPATION).

✓ Drink at least 8–10 glasses of pure spring water daily.
✓ Eat foods high in fiber, including plenty of fresh fruits and vegetables, whole grains, and legumes.

And Try This!

Try adding 3–4 tablespoons of oat bran fiber to juice, cereals, and baked goods. This not only promotes regularity, but also protects the appendix.

Did You Know?

In a study comparing the diets of 135 young people with appendicitis and 212 without it, Dr. Jean Brender, at the Audie Murphy Veterans Administration Hospital in San Antonio, Texas, disclosed that diets low in fiber, particularly whole grains, placed these individuals at twice the risk of an appendicitis attack. Fiber speeds up the transit time of wastes so that there's no pressure on the appendix. Research indicates that vegetarians, who eat lots of fiber, rarely develop appendicitis.

Arrhythmias (Irregular Heartbeats)

Arrhythmias can occur in different forms, but all are disruptions in normal heartbeat patterns due to the heart's electrical system cells not functioning properly. Common examples include heart palpitations (pounding heartbeats), ectopic beats (skipped heartbeats), and fibrillations (heart twitches).

Recognizing Arrhythmias

Arrhythmias range from mild to severe—from a skipped beat on rare occasions to frequent irregularities that make you light-headed, dizzy, weak, short of breath, and subject to heavy chest pain.

Warning: Always contact your doctor or get to a hospital immediately upon experiencing severe chest pain.

What Are the Causes of Arrhythmias?

- Stress
- Alcohol abuse
- Caffeine
- Smoking
- Heart valve defects
- Kidney disease
- Hyperthyroidism
- Nutritional deficiencies (especially magnesium and taurine)
- Drugs (especially diuretics since they can flush away magnesium, potassium, and manganese, minerals essential to the heart remaining on beat)

What You Can Take

Nutrients

Name	Dosage	Benefits
Coenzyme Q-10	50 mg twice daily	Stabilizes heart rhythm and helps relieve congestive heart failure.
Magnesium	400–800 mg daily	Corrects arrhythmias.
Omega-3 oils	500 mg softgels three times daily	Corrects arrhythmias.
Taurine	1–3 g daily	An enabler to magnesium. Can also help stabilize hearth rhythm on its own.

Herbs

Name	Dosage	Benefits
Astragalus	400 mg daily after breakfast and lunch	Strengthens heart muscles, making them more likely to contract and rest at proper intervals.

Name	Dosage	Benefits
Hawthorn	100 mg after each meal	Strengthens heartbeat.
	Warning: Not to be used if you are taking digitalis medications.	

What You Can Do

✓ Avoid smoking, alcohol, and caffeine—an approach that has been known for more than a century to minimize or eliminate arrhythmias.

✓ Relieve stress (*see* STRESS).

✓ Exercise regularly.

✓ Eat cold-water fish high in omega-3 oils (mackerel, sardines, salmon) twice a week.

✓ Eat foods high in the following nutrients:

- Magnesium, including blackstrap molasses, sunflower seeds, wheat germ, almonds, hazelnuts, Brazil nuts, pecans, walnuts, soy beans, soy lecithin, oats, barley, salmon, corn, avocados, bananas, cheese, tuna, and potatoes.
- Coenzyme Q-10, including salmon, sardines, mackerel, and spinach.

And Try This!

The amino acid L-carnitine, when taken orally at the rate of 2 g daily, can significantly improve conditions that are vital to heart health, including arrhythmias and even muscle damage. L-carnitine also appears to reduce the rate of recurring heart attacks and death from heart attack.

Did You Know?

Studies of Eskimos who are almost heart attack-free have focused attention on their eating cold-water fish. Omega-3 oil derived from fish has been found to correct arrhythmias, as reported in the *American Journal of Cardiology*.

Arthritis

The late, great George Burns was once asked if he'd ever had arthritis. "I got it when it first came out," he claimed. A stretch to be sure, as archaeologists have discovered that pre-historic Neanderthal man showed arthritic bones 40,000 to 100,000 years ago. So wouldn't you think, after all these centuries, researchers could come up with effective therapies for the two most widespread types of arthritis: *osteoarthritis*, a wearing away of cartilage between linking, weight-bearing bones, and *rheumatoid arthritis*, an inflammatory condition in which the immune system attacks its own body tissues? Some have—despite the tired thinking of many in the mainstream medical community who continue to tell us you can't cure it, but only deaden the pain.

Recognizing Arthritis

Osteoarthritis

- Usually occurs after age 40
- Pain and stiffness in the joints that generally develops over a period of several years
- Inflammation in later stages
- Muscle contractions
- Swollen joints
- Limited joint mobility

Rheumatoid Arthritis

- Can strike at all ages, and often occurs in children (juvenile rheumatoid arthritis)
- Pain and stiffness in the joints that is most pronounced in the morning
- Swollen joints
- Fatigue
- Fever

- Weight loss
- Anemia
- Night sweats
- Depression

What Are the Causes of Arthritis?

Osteoarthritis

Over and above wearing away of insulating cartilage between bones in osteoarthritis, there is a thickening of synovial tissues, a lubricated padding between bones and joint cavities that makes moving stiff, difficult, and painful. Major causes include:

- Obesity
- Sports and occupations that stress bones with unusual wear and tear
- Aging
- Food and environmental allergies
- Poor nutrition

Rheumatoid Arthritis

Although rheumatoid arthritis differs from osteoarthritis, it can start from the same roots—allergens, for instance. True allergic reactions involve the immune system, as do rheumatoid arthritis reactions, in a negative way. Here, the body's own immune system attacks the synovial system, a membrane that covers and insulates the joints and gives off synovial fluid, a lubricating liquid that permits adjoining bones to move painlessly against one another.

What You Can Take

Nutrients

Name	Dosage	Benefits
Vitamin A	10,000 IU daily	Essential to making and maintaining healthy cartilage.
Vitamin B-complex	100 mg daily	Helps relieve swelling associated with arthritis.
Vitamin C	1,000 mg three times daily	Helps repair cartilage tissue. Especially potent against rheumatoid arthritis when taken with manganese.
Vitamin E	800 IU daily	Stabilizes cell membranes, blocks the enzyme that causes a breakdown of cartilage, and sparks the making of cartilage.
Chondroitin sulfate	250-500 mg daily	Successful antiosteoarthritis agent.
Copper	2 mg daily	Strengthens connective tissue.
DHEA	50 mg daily *Warning:* Take only under the supervision of a physician. Do not take if you are at risk of hormone-related cancer.	Reduces pain and promotes joint flexibility.
Evening primrose oil	500 mg three times daily	High in essential fatty acids that help to relieve inflammation and pain.
Glucosamine sulfate	500 mg daily	Helps nullify pain and improve movement.
Manganese	15 mg daily	Promotes healthy bone growth.
Green-lipped mussel extract	Two 500 mg capsules daily	Effective anti-inflammatory.

Name	Dosage	Benefits
Methylsulfonyl-methane (MSM)	500 mg capsule twice daily	Renews permeability of hardened cell walls so that fluids can readily flow into cells, pick up toxins, and carry them off to enhance healing.
Niacinimide	1,000 mg three times daily	An anti-inflammatory especially useful in lessening knee pain.
Omega-3 oils	1,000 mg daily	High in essential fatty acids that help to relieve inflammation and pain.
S-adenosyl-methionine (SAMe)	400 mg twice daily for ten days to two weeks, then 300 mg twice daily for two weeks as maintenance	Anti-inflammatory that kills arthritic pain and helps in the rebuilding of cartilage.
Shark cartilage	Teaspoon of frozen sublingual product daily	Contains both chondroitin sulfate and glucosamine sulfate.
Zinc	30 mg daily	Deficiencies linked to arthritis.

Herbs

Name	Dosage	Benefits
Boswellia	150 mg three times daily	Reduces inflammation and helps build cartilage.
Bromelain	600 mg daily	An enzyme derived from pineapple that is a good anti-inflammatory, and promotes healing in the joints and muscles.
Curcumin (from turmeric)	400–1,200 mg daily	Powerful anti-inflammatory for arthritis.
Garlic (odorless)	2,500 mg capsules three times daily	Fights against free radicals, which can cause damage to the joints.

Name	Dosage	Benefits
Ginger	600 mg three times daily	Good all-purpose pain reliever.
Sea cucumber	1,000 mg daily	Diminishes pain and makes joints more flexible. Especially effective for arthritis of the hands.
Yucca	50 mg three times daily	Effective treatment for both major forms of arthritis by relieving swelling, stiffness, and pain.

Homeopathy

Name	Dosage	Benefits
Bryonia alba	6c every three hours	Relieves arthritis pain and inflammation.
Bryonia sulfur	6c every three hours	Relieves arthritis pain and inflammation.

What You Can Do

✓ Test for food and environmental allergies (*see* ALLERGIES).
✓ Avoid the following foods: eggplant, peppers, white potatoes, tomatoes, high-fat foods, sugar-rich foods, dairy products, red meat, alcohol, caffeine, citrus fruits, and salt.
✓ Increase consumption of the following foods: garlic, eggs, onions, asparagus, green leafy vegetables, nonacidic fresh fruits, whole grains, oatmeal, brown rice, fish, rye, and pineapple.
✓ Exercise regularly, but choose activities that do not put stress on affected joints.
✓ Avoid iron supplements, as iron has been known to increase painful swelling.
✓ Alternate hot/cold applications on inflamed joints.
✓ Take a hot bath or shower first thing in the morning.
✓ Maintain a healthy body weight (*see* OVERWEIGHT).

And Try This!

Try drinking kombucha tea. Rich in nutrients essential to maintaining strong connective tissue, it has been shown to increase mobility and alleviate pain in patients suffering from arthritis.

Did You Know?

In a survey involving 6,000 arthritis patients, Dr. Marshall Mandell, Medical Director of the New England Foundation for Allergic and Environmental Disease, found environmental and food allergens brought about allergic reactions in the joints of 85 percent of those tested.

Asthma

Asthma is dramatically on the rise (especially among children) and has reached what many consider epidemic levels in this country. More than 10 million Americans suffer from the condition. Some experts believe environmental pollution is to blame, but whatever the cause, deaths from asthma continue to mount at an alarming rate, largely because many susceptible people don't recognize the warning signs in time to take action.

Recognizing Asthma

Asthma causes the bronchial tubes (lung airways) to swell, spasm, and secrete thick mucus. The swelling narrows the airways and makes breathing difficult—sometimes impossible. Those having a first asthma attack are not always familiar with the symptoms. These can include:

- Wheezing (audible only when the airways are already half constricted)

- Coughing
- Tightness or congestion in the chest (sometimes pain)
- Shortness of breath
- Faster heart rate
- Feverish feeling
- Dryness of mouth

What Are the Causes of Asthma?

Any or every imaginable thing can bring on an asthma attack: an allergy, nutritional deficiency, respiratory infection, emotional disturbance, or strenuous exercise, to name a few of the most common. Allergies, however, tend to be the trigger more often than not in susceptible individuals. Some well-known examples are noted below.

Environmental Allergens

- Cigarette smoke
- Auto exhaust
- Molds, dusts, and pollens
- Animal dander
- Cockroaches
- Mites
- Pesticides
- Smog
- Lead
- Mercury and formaldehyde
- Natural gas odors
- Cleaning solvents
- Flouridated and chlorinated water

Highly Allergic Foods

- Milk and other dairy products
- Eggs
- Peanuts
- Pork
- Wheat
- Chocolate
- Corn
- Various spices

Allergens in/on Foods

- Antibiotics
- Hormones
- Tranquilizers

What You Can Take

Nutrients		
Name	**Dosage**	**Benefits**
Vitamin A	10,000 IU daily	Works with vitamin E to guard lungs against air pollution.
Vitamin B-complex	100 mg daily	Necessary for maintaining the biochemical balance of all B vitamins when supplementing with any single B vitamin individually.
Vitamin B_6	200 mg daily	Can reduce the frequency and severity of asthma attacks.
Vitamin B_{12}	1,000 mcg under the tongue daily	Protects against severe allergic reactions to sulfites.
Vitamin C	2,000 mg before workouts, 500 mg three times daily for minimal exercisers	Effective in preventing exercise-induced asthma attacks.
Vitamin E	400 IU daily	Powerful antioxidant that can help protect lungs from air pollution.
DHEA	5 mg daily *Warning:* Take only under the supervision of a physician. Do not take if you are at risk of hormone-related cancer.	Particularly useful for menopausal and postmenopausal women who develop asthma and are often low in DHEA.
Ginkgo biloba	120 mg daily	Enhances breathing and diminishes bronchial reactivity.
Hydrochloric acid	Formula consisting of 648 mg of betaine hydrochloride and 130 mg of pepsin	Helpful if there are digestive problems.
Magnesium	400 mg daily	Relaxes bronchial muscles.

Name	Dosage	Benefits
Omega-3	Two 500 mg capsules daily or fish twice weekly	Improves breathing.
Quercetin	500 mg before each meal	Blocks the release of anti-histamines and quenches free radical attacks that cause inflammation of the bronchial tubes.
Selenium	100–200 mcg daily	Protects against free radical damage brought on by environmental toxins.

Herbs

Name	Dosage	Benefits
Garlic (odorless)	One tablet or capsule after each meal	Strong anti-inflammatory agent.
Licorice root	200 mg three times daily	Loosens phlegm.
Tylophora asthmatica	120 mg daily	A key Indian herb in Ayurvedic medicine that blocks the release of histamines and other inflammatories.

Allergens in/on Foods (*cont'd*)

- Waxes
- Additives (artificial smoke, artificial colors, emulsifiers, thickeners, bleaches, antifoaming agents, and sweeteners, among the over 5,000 chemical additives authorized by the Food and Drug Administration)
- Sulfites (added to salad bar vegetables and fruit to keep them fresh-looking; and found in many brands of dried apricots, in processed potatoes, and in certain wines)

What You Can Do

✓ Test for food and environmental allergies (*see* ALLERGIES).

✓ Avoid allergens known to trigger asthmatic attacks (*see* "What Are the Causes of Asthma?").

✓ Eat a high-protein, low-carbohydrate diet that includes plenty of fresh fruits and vegetables.

✓ Avoid sugar and other refined carbohydrates.

✓ Eat five or six small meals throughout the day rather than the more traditional three large meals.

✓ Warm up slowly before all physical exercise. Don't overdo it.

✓ Minimize exposure to situations that ignite emotional disturbances.

✓ Use aspirin sparingly, if at all. It has been shown to trigger asthma attacks.

✓ Relieve stress (*see* STRESS).

And Try This!

Try drinking two cups of coffee quickly if you normally require the use of a bronchodilator to combat asthma attacks and find yourself caught without it. Coffee acts much the same way and can usually provide protection long enough to race to the nearest hospital for treatment.

Did You Know?

Certain off-the-wall conditions are responsible for asthma attacks, as illustrated by a study by George W. Ward, Jr., an associate professor of internal medicine at the University of Virginia. How about athlete's foot, jock itch, or ringworm? When he successfully treated such fungal infections among asthmatics, 66 percent of these patients reported a clearing up of their asthma symptoms!

Attention Deficit Disorder/Hyperactivity (ADD)

The usual treatment for hyperactive children—an easy out for physicians, parents, and teachers—is stimulants such as ritalin and amphetamines that curb their unruly conduct, calm them, and, supposedly, make them better able to learn. I say supposedly because reducing symptoms with ritalin fails to cope with hyperactivity's underlying causes and invites harmful side effects: chronic sleeplessness, tactile hallucinations (feeling a creeping sensation on the skin), and uncontrollable contraction of muscles. These can become even more pronounced when children quit the drug. *The Physician's Desk Reference* lists twenty-five horrendous examples, including anxiety, weight loss, slowing of growth, nausea, headaches, convulsions, hair loss, and grotesque conduct such as chewing fingers and nails until they bleed.

Thankfully, there are alternatives—though many in the pharmaceutical-dominated medical community would not have you know it!

Recognizing ADD

Boys outnumber girls 10 to 1 in diagnosed cases of ADD. Although the disorder may occur in adults, it is mainly associated with children. Any combination of the following symptoms may point to ADD:

- Self-destructive behavior
- Behavior disruptive to others
- Frequent mood swings
- Short attention span
- Inability to concentrate
- Problems sleeping
- Poor grades that don't reflect level of intelligence
- Learning disabilities
- Excessive fidgeting and nervousness
- Speech or hearing disorders
- Forgetfulness
- Tantrums

What Are the Causes of ADD?

ADD has been one of the most hotly debated (and controversial) health issues affecting children in recent years, both with respect to treatment and what causes the condition to begin with. Most experts agree that there may be many contributing factors, even in the same individual, and that each case needs to be looked at carefully when determining the source of the problem. Factors linked to ADD include the following:

- Food and environmental allergies
- Food additives
- Diet high in sugar and other refined carbohydrates
- Lack of dietary protein
- Caffeine
- Family history
- Lack of exercise
- Lead and other heavy metal poisoning
- Mother smoking while pregnant
- Learning disabilities
- Unstable home life

What You Can Do

- ✓ Beware the health hazards of ritalin.
- ✓ Test for food and environmental allergies (*see* ALLERGIES).
- ✓ Test (hair analysis) for toxic levels of heavy metals in the body.
- ✓ Test for learning disabilities.
- ✓ Exercise daily.
- ✓ Check labels and remove all foods that contain artificial flavorings, colors, preservatives, salicylates, nitrates, nitrites, phosphates, and aspartame.
- ✓ Avoid caffeine.
- ✓ Eat fresh, whole foods, including plenty of fruits and vegetables (other than those noted below).
- ✓ Avoid the following foods: soft drinks, bacon, butter, margarine, hot dogs, prepackaged meats, wheat, chocolate, milk, oranges, apples, tomatoes, peaches, berries, apricots, all processed foods, and especially sugar and other refined carbohydrates.

And Try This!

Try taking two to three 500 mg capsules of evening prim-rose oil daily. A major study of hyperactive children in the United States, Canada, United Kingdom, and South Africa found that more than two-thirds of those receiving such supplements experienced improvement or a complete recovery.

Did You Know?

A researcher in hyperactivity for more than 40 years, the late Dr. Ben Feingold, an allergist at Kaiser-Permanente Group Medical Center in San Francisco, discovered that additives in processed foods—some 5,000 artificial colorings, flavorings, and preservatives—were causing hyperactivity in his boy and girl patients, especially candy, baked goods, carbonated drinks, other bottled, canned foods, and packaged foods with a high content of sugar and refined flour. There were more than 1,200 cases in his files proving that food additives can bring on hyperactivity and that skipping them can reverse this condition. Dr. Feingold relieved their hyperactivity and, with parental approval, brought back this ailment with junk foods, to prove that he had found the root cause of this ailment. His remarkable healings inspired many of us in preventive or alternative medicine to use his methods with success.

Autism

Autism has been the subject of much speculation yet few answers. A brain disorder that is usually diagnosed in early childhood, estimates for the incidence of autism range from roughly 4 out of every 100,000 to 5 out of every 10,000 individuals born in the United States. Whether the actual incidence of autism has been increasing in recent years, or the disease has just become the subject of more media focus, many are now beginning to take a closer look at this puzzling condition.

Recognizing Autism

Since autism tends to be diagnosed before the age of 3, it is often first recognized by several of the following symptoms:

- Lack of interest in other people and physical surroundings
- Unresponsive to love and affection
- Sudden fits of hyperactivity
- Periods of prolonged silence and immobility
- Compulsive rocking behavior
- Poor speech development
- Various learning disabilities

What Are the Causes of Autism?

There is no single known cause of autism. Studies involving twins suggest there may be genetic factors involved, but such findings are not definitive. Others have argued that, at least in some cases, autism may be the result of adverse reactions to vaccines. Additional suspects include the following:

- Food and environmental allergies
- Nutritional deficiencies (especially vitamin B_6 and magnesium)

What You Can Take

Nutrients

Name	Dosage	Benefits
Vitamin B_6	3.5 to nearly 100 mg daily for every 2.2 pounds of body weight *Warning:* Have a nutrition-oriented doctor help you monitor a dosage this high to be safe.	Deficiencies linked to autism.
Dimethylglycine (DMG)	120–180 mg daily.	Improves mood, attention span, and can help limit the number of tantrums.

Name	Dosage	Benefits
Magnesium	1,000 mg daily. Combine with 50 mg three times daily of vitamin B$_6$ *Warning:* Have a nutrition-oriented doctor help you monitor dosage this high to be safe.	Deficiencies linked to autism.

Herbs

Name	Dosage	Benefits
Ginkgo biloba	Capsule form as directed on label	Increases blood flow to the brain.

- Fetal alcohol syndrome
- Viral infections during pregnancy of the mother
- Yeast overgrowth
- Gastrointestinal disorders
- Toxic levels of lead and other heavy metals in the blood

What You Can Do

✓ Eliminate processed foods with chemical additives and a high content of sugar and refined carbohydrates.

✓ Test for food and environmental allergies (*see* ALLERGIES).

✓ Test (hair analysis) for toxic levels of heavy metals in the body.

✓ Eat foods high in the following nutrients:
  - Vitamin B$_6$, including brewer's yeast, brown rice, whole wheat, royal jelly, soybeans, rye, lentils, sunflower seeds, alfalfa, salmon, wheat germ, tuna, bran, walnuts, cashews, peanuts, peas, liver, avocados, beans, turkey, oats, chicken, halibut, lamb, and bananas.
  - Magnesium, including blackstrap molasses, sunflower seeds, wheat germ, almonds, hazelnuts, Brazil nuts, pecans, walnuts, soybeans, soy lecithin, oats, barley, salmon, corn, avocados, bananas, cheese, tuna, and potatoes.

✓ Seek out special educational options for autistic children.

And Try This!

Try chelation therapy, a safe and effective means of ridding the body of heavy toxic metals such as lead and mercury. Chelation therapy can be performed either orally or intravenously. Please consult with a physician trained in this practice, as it requires close medical supervision.

Did You Know?

According to Bernard Rimland, Ph.D., the father of an autistic child and director of the Autism Research Institute in San Diego, studies indicate that between 30 to 60 percent of autistic patients tested experience significant improvements following supplementation with high doses of vitamin B_6 and magnesium.

Back Pain

Physiologists often claim that human beings pay for their upright posture with many painful back problems. Yet it wouldn't be socially acceptable or practical to walk on all fours. So the solutions have to come within your and my limitations.

Unlike our upright distant ancestors who walked and ran to hunt and gather, and more recent ancestors who planted, watered, and harvested—or made things standing at a workbench—we work mainly while sitting at workplaces or desks or in cars, trucks, or busses. So back and stomach muscles that hold our spine in place are weak.

Recognizing Back Problems

A telltale symptom is unceasing aching along the spine, pain in the neck, and back—upper or lower—particularly when bending to lift or taking part in strenuous movements. Another is lower back pain when standing.

What Are the Causes of Back Pain?

Causes are weak or stressed back or abdominal muscles or an X-ray-revealed herniated disk, a bulge in one of the cushion-like shock absorbers that separates the pile of 24 vertebrae. This presses against a nerve, which causes pain.

Underlying are these causes:

- Poor diet
- Weak bones
- Lack of physical exercise
- Poor posture
- Wrong lifting techniques
- Strain of pregnancy

What You Can Take

Nutrients

Name	Dosage	Benefits
Vitamin C	1,000 mg daily	Strengthens bones and cartilage.
Vitamin D	400 IU daily	Enhances calcium absorption.
Calcium	600 mg daily before bedtime	Strengthens bones.
Magnesium	400 mg daily	Works with calcium to strengthen bones.
Manganese	40 mg twice daily	Vital to bone and cartilage integrity.
Boron	2–4 mg daily	Helpful in bone rebuilding.
Bromelain	500 mg three times daily	Reduces inflammation and pain.
Glucosamine sulfate	500 mg after each meal	Strengthens cartilage and spinal disks.
Omega-3 oils	500 mg softgel daily	Lessens pain and inflammation.

Herbs

Name	Dosage	Benefits
White willow extract	2 ml three times daily	Relieves pain like aspirin.

What You Can Do

✓ Exercise regularly for muscle flexibility and strength to prevent back pain. Walking and swimming are best bets.

✓ Take *only* one or two days of bed rest for excruciating pain, then slowly become active.

✓ Use hot water bag or heating pad on the pain site.

✓ Ice bag on pain site—5–10 minutes at a time—often helps inflammation.

✓ Do gentle stretches to speed healing.

✓ Add calcium-containing foods to your diet—milk, if you're not allergic or intolerant, broccoli, sardines, salmon, kale, pinto beans, and almonds.

✓ Stop smoking to accelerate healing.

✓ Improve posture.

✓ Put aside tight-fitting slacks in favor of loose-fitting garments that permit free and normal movement.

✓ Wear high heels only for special occasions.

✓ Bend your knees when lifting and keep lifted object as near to the body as possible.

✓ Lift first, then turn your body when placing a heavy object.

✓ Take frequent breaks when sitting at work.

✓ Support lower back when seated.

✓ Sleep on a firm mattress on your side or back, never on your belly.

✓ See your doctor when pain is accompanied by fever and vomiting.

✓ Get a second opinion when surgery is suggested.

And Try This!

This simple exercise often helps my patients. Lie down and draw your knees up to your chest. Then stretch and relax. Repeat this several times unless pain strikes. Try this sequence three times daily.

Did You Know?

It is natural to resist regular exercise when your back hurts, but this can be harmful, as research with 187 back pain patients at two universities in England demonstrated. Those who exercised regularly with a physiotherapist relieved their pain more quickly than nonexercisers and were able to resume normal activities faster.

Bad Breath (Halitosis)

Between patients, I had just read a newspaper article about an Egyptian pyramid being closed to tourists because their breath had begun to erode the stone. By strange coincidence my next patient, a middle-aged woman, had a problem with breath—bad breath that belonged to her husband. Nearly in tears, she told me, "Doctor, his breath is so foul it would peel off the wallpaper. No mouthwash can mask it. I can't sleep with him. Forget sex! Others in his office complain about him. I'm afraid he'll be fired." Breath that bad starts way down in the intestines. Incompletely digested food putrifies there and, added to constipation and impacted waste matter, causes odoriferous breath.

Recognizing Bad Breath

If you can smell your own bad breath, so can others!

What Are the Causes of Bad Breath?

- Poor dental hygiene
- Constipation
- Indigestion
- Sinus infections
- Diabetes
- Diet high in sugar and other refined carbohydrates
- Stress
- Smoking
- Coffee
- Alcohol
- Spicy foods

What You Can Take

Nutrients

Name	Dosage	Benefits
Vitamin B-complex	100 mg daily	Aids digestion.
Vitamin C	500 mg three times daily	Helps firm up spongy gums where food can get trapped.
Hydrochloric acid	One capsule containing 650 mg of betaine hydrochloride and 130 mg of pepsin with each meal	Aids digestion.

What You Can Do

✓ Have a Heidelberg test to determine the amount of hydrochloric acid being secreted in the stomach.

✓ Brush gums and tongue, and floss (if possible) after every meal.

✓ Drink at least 8–10 glass of pure spring water daily.

✓ Chew parsley, fragrant basil, mint, rosemary, thyme, or wintergreen following meals.

✓ Avoid sugar and other refined carbohydrates.

✓ Avoid obvious odor-inducing foods such as garlic, onions, coffee, and anchovies.

✓ Add fiber to the diet to increase regularity (*see* CONSTIPATION).

✓ Eat 16 ounces of plain yogurt with active cultures daily, in three divided portions before meals.

✓ Eat plenty of fresh, raw fruits and vegetables.

✓ Eat foods high in vitamin C, including rose hips, acerola cherries, guavas, black currants, red peppers, oranges, grapefruit and other citrus fruits, cabbage, papayas, cantaloupe, and tomatoes.

And Try This!

Try gargling with 1 tablespoon of chlorophyll mixed in a glass of spring water. It may just work wonders!

Did You Know?

An authority on dental problems, Dr. Frederick M. Kraus regards mouthwashes as a short-term cover-up for bad breath and a hazard if used continually. Mouthwashes designed to kill harmful bacteria also kill helpful microorganisms. This upsets nature's balance, removing the protection of friendly bacteria. Some mouthwashes are even toxic, according to Dr. Kraus. Others contain antibiotics that can cause allergies.

Bedsores

An ailment such as bedsores may sound trivial to someone who has never been bedridden for long periods of time. Not true! Bedsores among paraplegics—those paralyzed from the hips down—have caused an estimated 10 percent rate of deaths. Such sores are foul-smelling, deep, supersized, and bleed so profusely that precious blood, blood protein, and other key nutrients are lost. Resulting anemia, overwhelming fatigue, weakened immune resistance, and depression often gang up and make the victim vulnerable to devastating infectious diseases.

Recognizing Bedsores

Sometimes also referred to as pressure sores, bedsores can be extremely painful and are most commonly found on the following areas of the body:

- Buttocks
- Shoulders
- Hips
- Lower back
- Heels

What Are the Causes of Bedsores?

Limited in movement, bedridden patients experience constant pressure from hard bone on soft tissue and reduced circulation in certain areas, starving and killing cells, and causing ulcers that aggravate pain and soreness. Those suffering from bedsores are often deficient in important nutrients as well, including vitamin C, vitamin A, and zinc.

What You Can Take

Nutrients

Name	Dosage	Benefits
Vitamin A	25,000–50,000 IU daily *Warning:* Pregnant and pregnancy-eligible women should take no more than 10,000 IU daily.	Essential for skin healing.
Vitamin C	500 mg three times daily	Excellent for wound healing.
Flavonoids	250 mg (200 mg from citrus and 50 mg from buckwheat) three times daily	Works with vitamin C to promote wound healing.
Zinc	25–50 mg daily plus 2 mg of copper to maintain proper zinc-copper ratio	Promotes healing in general, especially when taken with vitamin A.

What You Can Do

✓ Change positions frequently (at least every few hours).
✓ Gently massage bedsore areas to increase blood circulation.
✓ Apply aloe vera gel and marigold comfrey ointments to bedsores.

✓ Drink at least 8–10 glasses of pure spring water daily.
✓ Keep skin dry.
✓ Eat foods high in the following nutrients:
  - Proteins, including eggs, meat, fish, and fowl.
  - Vitamin A, including eggs, milk, cheese, cream, butter, yogurt, salmon, bass, halibut, mackerel, herring, whitefish, sardines, tuna, clams, shrimp, beef, chicken, pistachios, pecans, walnuts, lentils, and soybeans.
  - Vitamin C, including rose hips, acerola cherries, guavas, black currants, red peppers, oranges, grapefruit and other citrus fruits, cabbage, papayas, cantaloupe, and tomatoes.
  - Zinc, including seafood, sardines, oysters, soybeans, soy lecithin, kelp, legumes, meats, liver, eggs, brewer's yeast, mushrooms, poultry, whole grains, and pumpkin and sunflower seeds.

And Try This!

Try wearing cotton clothes that fit loosely. They allow the skin to breathe and prevent sores from forming due to rough seams pressing or rubbing against vulnerable areas of the body.

Did You Know?

There are mechanical apparatuses that many hospitals use to take the pressure off bedsores: waterbeds that cause a shifting of weight and an improvement of blood circulation, supersoft padding to be put under patients' bedsore areas, as well as foam "egg crate" sheets or mattresses with peaks and valleys. These can be bought or rented for the home at hospital supply stores.

Bedwetting

Urologists and pediatricians tell me that most children overcome bedwetting by the time they are five years old. Unfortunately, some don't make it until entering their teens (if not later) and, consequently, endure years of humiliation and punishment. In almost every case it is not their fault.

What Are the Causes of Bedwetting?

- A smaller than normal bladder
- Food and environmental allergies
- Drinking too many liquids before bedtime
- Magnesium deficiency
- Cystitis
- Stress

What You Can Take

Nutrients

Name	Dosage	Benefits
Magnesium	250 mg tablet daily for a minimum of one month	Deficiencies linked to bedwetting.
Multivitamin and mineral complex	As directed on label	Maintenance dose of magnesium to prevent deficiencies.

What You Can Do

- ✓ Test for food and environmental allergies (*see* ALLERGIES).
- ✓ Be aware that chocolate, eggs, milk, processed foods, and food additives are among the common allergens that cause bladder hypersensitivity.
- ✓ Avoid fluids after four in the afternoon, except in emergencies.

✓ Empty bladder before bed.

✓ Massage lower back with gentle finger and palm pressure.

✓ Add brown rice, millet, fresh vegetables, fresh diluted carrot juice, and small amounts of cherry juice to the diet.

✓ Eat foods rich in magnesium, including sunflower seeds, almonds, hazelnuts, salmon, cheeses, tuna, turkey, halibut, liver, wheat germ, and blackstrap molasses.

✓ Withhold punishment. It only humiliates the child. Compliment or reward the child for a night without bedwetting instead.

✓ Attempt to limit the child's anxiety about the problem without giving the impression that it is all right.

And Try This!

Try having the child drink a daily cup of warm tea made from a tablespoon of marjoram leaf. You can also mix the same amount in a sandwich or salads.

Did You Know?

Some years ago, Dr. John W. Gerard, professor of pediatrics at the University of Saskatchewan, investigated the problem with 223 nonbedwetters and 75 bedwetters. He amazed the medical profession with his announcement that bladders of bedwetters were almost half the size of those of nonbedwetters. And the bladder capacity of youngsters who lost control by night and day was the smallest of the small.

Bell's Palsy

Patients stricken with Bell's Palsy, a paralysis of one side of the face, often imagine they have any of several disorders: lockjaw, an infected or abscessed tooth, or even a stroke. The good news is that, unlike those conditions, Bell's Palsy almost always goes away by itself. However, it can drag on for weeks, sometimes months. Fortunately, certain measures can be taken to speed its departure.

Recognizing Bell's Palsy

- Facial muscles and nerves become swollen and rigid
- Swelling causes the nerves to be compressed against tissue
- Pain (sometimes excruciating)
- Numbness
- Can become difficult to talk or eat

What Are the Causes of Bell's Palsy?

As I have observed many times in my decades of practice, Bell's Palsy can be brought about by many factors, all of them stressors of one kind or another:

- Chicken pox or shingles virus
- Cold or flu
- Severe infection
- Menstrual cycle
- Infected tooth
- Cold burst of air to the face
- Stress

What You Can Take

Nutrients

Name	Dosage	Benefits
Vitamin A	20,000 IU daily *Warning:* Pregnant and pregnancy-eligible women should not take more than 10,000 IU daily.	Works with zinc to help reduce swelling and encourage healing.
Vitamin B-complex	100 mg daily	Helps relieve inflamed nerves.
Vitamin C	1,000–2,000 mg three times daily	Potent anti-inflammatory that fights bacterial infections.

Name	Dosage	Benefits
Vitamin E	800 IU daily	Powerful antioxidant that provides relief to inflamed nerves.
Selenium	200 mcg daily	Helps relieve swelling.
Zinc	15 mg daily	Works with vitamin A to reduce swelling and encourage healing.

Herbs		
Name	Dosage	Benefits
Aged garlic extract	Six squirts from a squeezable plastic container in a half glass of water three times daily	Highly effective against bacterial infections.

What You Can Do

✓ Work to relieve stress (*see* STRESS).
✓ Eat foods high in the following nutrients:
  • Vitamin A, including eggs, milk, cheese, cream, butter, yogurt, salmon, bass, halibut, mackerel, herring, whitefish, sardines, tuna, clams, shrimp, beef, chicken, pistachios, pecans, walnuts, lentils, and soybeans.
  • Vitamin C, including rose hips, acerola cherries, guavas, black currants, red peppers, oranges, grapefruit and other citrus fruits, cabbage, papayas, cantaloupe, and tomatoes.
  • Vitamin E, including sunflower seeds, whole wheat, peanuts, cashews, almonds, walnuts, corn oil, soy oil, soy lecithin, spinach, asparagus, broccoli, butter oats, and avocados.
  • Selenium, including Brazil nuts, fish, organ meats, whole grains, eggs, cabbage, corn, peas, onions, garlic, chicken, beets, barley, and tomatoes.
  • Zinc, including seafood, sardines, oysters, soybeans,

soy lecithin, kelp, legumes, meats, liver, eggs, brewer's yeast, mushrooms, poultry, whole grains, and pumpkin and sunflower seeds.

And Try This!

Try taking the homeopathic remedy causticum. A dose of 30c taken four times daily for three days has brought relief to a number of my Bell's Palsy patients in pain.

Did You Know?

Nerves—inflamed or not—are under constant attack by free radicals. Dr. Bruce Ames, a molecular biologist at the University of California at Berkeley, estimates that every cell in the body is hit by free radicals 10,000 times daily. These are molecular muggers, molecules that have lost an electron and attack neighboring molecules, forcibly stealing an electron. This causes a chain reaction that antioxidants such as vitamins A, C, E, and the minerals selenium and zinc can stop.

Beriberi

Common opinion holds that the disease beriberi exists only in the Far East in populations that live mainly on polished rice, whose major nutrient, vitamin B_1 (thiamine), has been milled away. Unfortunately, common opinion is often uncommonly wrong. Subclinical beriberi is flourishing in the United States in some alcoholics, some pregnant women, in many stressed-out individuals, hyperthyroid patients, elderly people who don't metabolize food efficiently, and those who try to live on highly processed foods. The word *beriberi* comes from a Philippine expression, "I can't. I can't." And believe me, those with full-blown beriberi can't do much physically or mentally until they add vitamin B_1 to their diets.

Recognizing Beriberi

Members of those groups noted above (particularly alcoholics) are most at risk for beriberi. Typical symptoms include:

- Appetite loss
- Confusion
- Constipation
- Diarrhea
- Lack of coordination
- Edema (fluid retention)

- Extreme fatigue
- Hair-trigger temper
- Heart failure
- Nervousness
- Paralysis
- Poor memory

What Are the Causes of Beriberi?

Beriberi is caused by a deficiency in vitamin B_1 (thiamine). Factors that can contribute to such a deficiency include the following:

- Alcohol abuse
- Diet high in processed foods
- Pregnancy
- Stress

- Hyperthyroidism
- Infection
- Frequent use of antacids and diuretics

What You Can Take

Nutrients

Name	Dosage	Benefits
Vitamin B-complex	100 mg daily	Reverses and prevents vitamin B_1 deficiency.
Vitamin C	500 mg three times daily	Required for optimal absorption of B vitamins.
Vitamin E	400 IU daily	Deficiencies often found in those with beriberi.
Multivitamin and mineral complex	As directed on label	Prevents general deficiencies associated with beriberi.

What You Can Do

✓ Avoid alcohol.
✓ Avoid the use of antacids and diuretics.
✓ Avoid sugar and other refined carbohydrates.
✓ Avoid processed foods.
✓ Avoid drinking liquids during meals, as it stifles absorption of B vitamins.
✓ Work to relieve stress (*see* STRESS).
✓ Eat foods high in the following nutrients:
   - Vitamin B_1, including brown rice, whole wheat grains, wheat germ, beans, nuts, oats, liver, yogurt, and raw fruits and vegetables.
   - Vitamin C, including rose hips, acerola cherries, guavas, black currants, red peppers, oranges, grapefruit and other citrus fruits, cabbage, papayas, cantaloupe, and tomatoes.
   - Vitamin E, including sunflower seeds, whole wheat, peanuts, cashews, almonds, walnuts, corn oil, soy oil, soy lecithin, spinach, asparagus, broccoli, oats, and avocados.

And Try This!

Try the following daily regimen: at least 4 ounces of protein such as an egg or a small piece of meat, fish, or poultry; a dinner salad and fresh fruit or vegetable with each meal; multivitamin tablet, multi-mineral tablet, and a 100 mg vitamin B-complex tablet.

Did You Know?

Some years ago, a proposal was made to add vitamin B_1 to alcohol. This recommendation went through nutrition committee after committee and was finally tabled. One theory as to why is that it would only encourage alcoholics to continue overdrinking.

Bronchitis

A severe inflammation and/or blocking of the bronchi (air tubes in the lungs), bronchitis is one ailment that can hang on as tenaciously as a bulldog. Bronchitis occurs in one of two forms: acute or chronic. The difference is generally causal in nature, with acute bronchitis being the less serious condition of the two. Still, acute bronchitis can last several weeks and may result in pneumonia if not attended to. Chronic bronchitis can eventually lead to serious heart problems.

Recognizing Bronchitis

- Phlegm-producing, frequent, often painful cough
- Fever up to 100° F
- Difficulty breathing
- Harsh sounds when breathing
- Chest pain
- Sore throat
- Chills

What Are the Causes of Bronchitis?

Acute bronchitis is most often the result of an infection such as a cold or the flu. Chronic bronchitis is generally caused by an irritant to the lungs. Common examples include tobacco smoke, dust, allergies, and various forms of air pollution.

What You Can Take

Nutrients

Name	Dosage	Benefits
Vitamin A	20,000 IU daily for up to thirty days *Warning:* Pregnant and pregnancy-eligible women should take no more than 10,000 IU daily.	Promotes healing of inflamed mucus membranes and strengthens immune system.

Name	Dosage	Benefits
Vitamin C	1,000 mg three times daily	Boosts immunity and contributes to sound collagen in the windpipe and bronchial mucus linings for healing.
Vitamin E	400 IU daily	Powerful antioxidant that can help protect lungs from air pollution.
N-acetylcysteine (NAC)	250 mg three to four times daily	Thins mucus, making it more easily expelled.
Zinc	30 mg daily	Works together with vitamin A for healing of mucus membranes and other tissue.

Herbs

Name	Dosage	Benefits
Astragalus	200 mg three times daily	Reduces symptoms associated with chronic bronchitis.

What You Can Do

✓ Don't smoke and avoid secondhand smoke.
✓ Avoid pollution by staying indoors during smog alerts.
✓ Do not use sprays (outdoor and indoor) for cleaning, deodorizing, or insect-repelling.
✓ Avoid dairy products, as they increase mucus formation.
✓ Get plenty of rest when first contracting the condition.
✓ Apply heat to chest and back before bed.
✓ Drink at least 8–10 glasses of pure spring water daily.
✓ Eat foods high in the following nutrients:
  • Vitamin A, including eggs, salmon, bass, halibut, mackerel, herring, whitefish, sardines, tuna, clams, shrimp, beef, chicken, pistachios, pecans, walnuts, lentils, and soybeans.
  • Vitamin C, including rose hips, acerola cherries, guavas, black currants, red peppers, oranges, grape-

fruit and other citrus fruits, cabbage, papayas, cantaloupe, and tomatoes.
- Vitamin E, including sunflower seeds, whole wheat, peanuts, cashews, almonds, walnuts, corn oil, soy oil, soy lecithin, spinach, asparagus, broccoli, oats, and avocados.
- Zinc, including seafood, sardines, oysters, soybeans, soy lecithin, kelp, legumes, meats, liver, eggs, brewer's yeast, mushrooms, poultry, whole grains, and pumpkin and sunflower seeds.

And Try This!

Try drinking a quarter to half a cup of horehound tea three times daily. It helps to thin and release mucus that accumulates in patients with bronchitis.

Did You Know?

It is a serious self-treatment mistake to take antihistamines or decongestants or antibiotics for bronchitis. Antihistamines and decongestants won't relieve conditions in the windpipes or bronchial tubes, may dry their mucus linings, and make the mucus so thick that it can be difficult and painful to cough up. Likewise, antibiotics don't usually help (most bronchitis is not caused by bacterial infection), and they could hurt by killing off friendly microorganisms and contribute to making certain bacteria more antibiotic-resistant.

Brown Spots (Aging Spots, Liver Spots)

While editor of *Let's Live* magazine, Jim Scheer received an unusual letter from a reader about how she coped with brown spots on her hands—one that he couldn't print. This elderly lady liberally soaped her hands and then, using a moderately stiff brush, brushed the spots for several minutes daily. She claimed that, after she followed this special protocol for a few weeks, the brown spots disappeared. Knowing that the skin of middle-aged to elderly individuals becomes thinner, more easily bruised, and therefore, subject to infection, Jim thought better of running the letter.

Recognizing Brown Spots

Brown spots, or aging or liver spots, as they are commonly known, can generally be seen first on the face, neck, and hands. While harmless in their own right, they may be a visible indication of further deterioration going on inside the body.

What Are the Causes of Brown Spots?

When oxygen interacts with highly unsaturated fats (polyunsaturates), free radicals (peroxides) are formed. These damaged cells leave behind wastes called lipofuscin, not only in the skin, but also in organs of the body. A buildup of this lipofuscin is what creates the spots. Factors that contribute to this buildup include:

- Excessive sun exposure
- Lack of exercise
- Liver damage
- Nutritional deficiencies (especially vitamins C and E)

What You Can Take

Nutrients

Name	Dosage	Benefits
Vitamin C	1,000 mg three times daily	Helps to restore vitamin E that has been lost in the fight against free radicals.
Vitamin E	1,200 IU daily	Powerful antioxidant that attacks free radicals.
Grape seed or pine bark extract	100 mg twice daily	Protects vitamin C.

What You Can Do

✓ Exercise daily (I suggest a 30-minute walk).
✓ Drink at least 8–10 glasses of pure spring water daily.
✓ Apply retinoic acid, a metabolite of vitamin A, to brown spots daily.
✓ Avoid caffeine.
✓ Avoid sugar and other refined carbohydrates.
✓ Don't smoke.
✓ Limit sun exposure.
✓ Eat a fresh fruit or vegetable with every meal.
✓ Eat foods high in the following nutrients:
  • Vitamin C, including rose hips, acerola cherries, guavas, black currants, red peppers, oranges, grapefruit and other citrus fruits, cabbage, papayas, cantaloupe, and tomatoes.
  • Vitamin E, including sunflower seeds, whole wheat, peanuts, cashews, almonds, walnuts, corn oil, soy oil, soy lecithin, spinach, asparagus, broccoli, oats, and avocados.

And Try This!

You might want to try the anti-brown spots formula of H. L. Newbold, M.D., of New York City: eliminating processed foods and taking vitamins C and E and the minerals zinc and selenium, and essential fatty acids. My version of the Newbold formula also calls for junking junk foods and taking 1,500 mg of vitamin C three times daily, 800 IU of vitamin E, 30 mg of zinc, and 200 mcg of selenium daily, plus at least 8–9 glasses of water, and walking for 30 minutes daily. It has helped lessen the number of brown spots and their color in a number of my patients.

Did You Know?

Results of a study at the University of Michigan Medical Center found that when retinoic acid, a metabolite of vitamin A, was dabbed on brown spots daily, the spots lightened up noticeably after just 1 month. Following 10 months of such treatment, the brown spots did not return for 6 months in 6 of the 7 patients studied.

Bruising

The new patient was embarrassed. Middle-aged, slightly overweight, and depressed, she drew back a sleeve of her plain, white blouse. Her fleshy arm was blotched with red bruises, some the size of silver dollars. Her legs were covered with them, too. As if anticipating my first thought, she said, "No one has hurt me, Doctor. These are spontaneous." Spontaneous until we probed a little further. Turns out she'd been taking an aspirin a day to prevent a heart attack based on the advice of a radio health commentator. Mystery solved!

Recognizing Bruising

Bruises begin as painful red blotches under the skin, gradually becoming a darker blue/black, before fading to more of a yellow color as they heal. Bruises vary in size and intensity depending on the source of the injury.

What Are the Causes of Bruising?

Bruises are generally the result of a blow to a specific area of the body, like bumping into something or perhaps a fall. Capillaries burst and spill blood under the skin. Everyone's had them, but some are more prone to easy bruising than others. Factors that can contribute to a tendency to bruise easily include the following:

- Regular use of aspirin (keeps blood from clotting too readily)
- Vitamin C deficiency
- Smoking
- Overweight
- Poor nutrition

What You Can Take

Nutrients

Name	Dosage	Benefits
Vitamin B-complex	100 mg daily	Promotes the production of mature blood platelets to assure normal clotting.
Vitamin C	500 mg three times daily	Important to the synthesis of collagen.
Acidophilus (probiotics)	Three 500 mg capsules daily	Implants friendly bacteria in the colon in order to help synthesize vitamin K, essential to blood clotting.
Bioflavonoids	200 mg to every 500 mg of vitamin C	Works with vitamin C to strengthen the walls of capillaries.

What You Can Do

✓ Avoid taking daily aspirin if you bruise easily.
✓ Gently smooth aloe vera gel on the red blotches.
✓ Apply an ice pack to bruised area quickly after injury.
✓ Eat a pint of cultured, unsweetened yogurt daily.
✓ Eat plenty of whole grains and fresh fruits and vegetables.
✓ Eat foods high in vitamin C, including rose hips, acerola cherries, guavas, black currants, red peppers, oranges, grapefruit and other citrus fruits, cabbage, papayas, cantaloupe, and tomatoes.

And Try This!

Try an ice bag on bruises or ice in a wash cloth—never ice directly on the skin—for 10 minutes of every hour for 24 hours. This treatment has caused black and blue coloring and swelling on my patients' skin to disappear quickly.

Did You Know?

For many decades trainers of professional and college contact sports teams—football, soccer, basketball—have put players on pregame vitamin C with bioflavonoids (usually 500 to 1,000 mg) to strengthen the walls of their capillaries and prevent or reduce bruising.

Bruxism (Teeth Grinding)

Bruxism is a fancy medical term for grinding your teeth. And you may be doing so without even knowing it, as it usually occurs during sleep.

Recognizing Bruxism

A dentist will most often be the first one to spot the condition. Symptoms of bruxism may include:

- Loose teeth
- Receding gums
- Misaligned bite
- Tooth loss

What Are the Causes of Bruxism?

- Stress and anxiety
- Sensitive teeth
- Fluctuating blood sugar levels
- Diet high in sugar and other refined carbohydrates

What You Can Take

Nutrients		
Name	**Dosage**	**Benefits**
Vitamin B-complex	100 mg daily	Contains pantothenic acid, a proven stress fighter.
Calcium citrate	500–1,000 mg daily	Helps control involuntary muscle movements.

What You Can Do

✓ Be alert for grinding teeth.
✓ Work to relieve stress (*see* STRESS).
✓ Avoid sugar and other refined carbohydrates.
✓ Avoid alcohol.
✓ Consult with your dentist about devices that can be worn over the teeth at night until the problem is corrected.

And Try This!

Try having someone observe you in your sleep. You may be grinding your teeth, even though your dentist has not yet noticed any symptoms.

Did You Know?

When teeth are loose from bruxism, you can tighten them within 10 days by going on a diet low in sugar and other refined carbohydrates.

Burns

Burns are grouped into one of three types: first, second, and third degree. Almost everyone has experienced first-degree burns, reddening of the skin. Second-degree burns are less common and involve blistering and some skin destruction. Third-degree burns often destroy the full thickness of the skin and underlying tissues, sometimes reaching the bone. When burns are severe, shock can occur. Body fluids—blood and lymph—and electrolytes rush to the damaged area. Blood pressure almost shuts down, as a protective measure. Although blood vessels constrict, much blood may escape through a skin break, making a transfusion necessary.

Recognizing Burns

- *First-degree* burns injure only the skin's outer layer. Redness and pain occur. Sunburn is a good example.
- *Second-degree* burns carry the same symptoms as first-degree burns, but affect underlying layers of the skin. Blistering may also occur and the pain is more intense.
- *Third-degree* burns cause severe damage to both the outer and inner layers of the skin and can destroy surrounding tissue (including muscle). Skin may appear several different colors ranging from red to white to black. The pain is often less than in first- or second-degree burns because nerve tissue has been damaged.

Warning: Seek immediate medical attention for severe burns. Never attempt to treat a third-degree burn yourself.

What Are the Causes of Burns?

Burns occur when the skin is heated more than 120° F, causing damage. Such heat can come from various sources, including fire, flat irons, torrid frying pans, barbecues, stoves, fireplaces, boiling water, sun exposure, radiation, and chemicals. Toddlers are especially attracted to objects that cause burns.

What You Can Take

Nutrients

Name	Dosage	Benefits
Vitamin A	25,000–50,000 IU daily for several weeks *Warning:* Pregnant or pregnancy-eligible women should take no more than 10,000 IU daily.	Immune enhancer that promotes rapid healing.
Vitamin C	250–500 mg three to four times daily	Boosts immune system and prevents infection. Required for growth of collagen and connective tissue.
Vitamin E	800 IU daily with vitamin E ointment applied several times daily	Powerful antioxidant and remedy against burns, both as a supplement and when administered topically.
Zinc	30 mg daily	Essential for healing burns, especially when taken with vitamin A.

Herbs

Name	Dosage	Benefits
Gotu kola extract	200 mg three times daily	Enhances growth of connective tissue.

What You Can Do

✓ Practice safety—especially with children—because prevention is still the best cure.

✓ Plunge victim's burned (first- and second-degree only) hand, arm, or leg into cold water at once. If burn occurs on areas of the body that cannot be submerged, wrap with cold towels.

✓ Dab aloe vera juice or gel on burns after the pain is gone.

✓ Apply calendula cream on burns to soothe them and promote healing.

✓ Adjust diet to contain more protein, increasing daily intake by 400 g.
✓ Drink at least 8–10 glasses of pure spring water daily to speed healing.
✓ Eat foods high in the following nutrients:
- Vitamin A, including eggs, milk, cheese, cream, butter, yogurt, salmon, bass, halibut, mackerel, herring, whitefish, sardines, tuna, clams, shrimp, beef, chicken, pistachios, pecans, walnuts, lentils, and soybeans.
- Vitamin C, including rose hips, acerola cherries, guavas, black currants, red peppers, oranges, grapefruit and other citrus fruits, cabbage, papayas, cantaloupe, and tomatoes.
- Vitamin E, including sunflower seeds, whole wheat, peanuts, cashews, almonds, walnuts, corn oil, soy oil, soy lecithin, spinach, asparagus, broccoli, oats, and avocados.
- Zinc, including seafood, sardines, oysters, soybeans, soy lecithin, kelp, legumes, meats, liver, eggs, brewer's yeast, mushrooms, poultry, whole grains, and pumpkin and sunflower seeds.

And Try This!

Try mixing a level teaspoon of vitamin C crystals with 2 cups of water to create a 1 percent vitamin C solution. Pour into an atomizer and spray on burns to relieve pain. You'll feel the results within minutes!

Did You Know?

It took a hydrogen bomb blast at the Bikini Atoll a generation ago to focus world attention on aloe vera as perhaps the greatest of all natural healers for burns. Despite the best efforts of the test crew to keep this south Pacific area clear of traffic for safety reasons, a Japanese fishing boat cleaved the waters not far from the Atoll. Occupants of the boat were covered with radioactive fallout. One fisherman died, and other crew members suffered what were thought to be fatal burns. In the book *Aloe, the Incredible,* Japanese biochemist Akira Yagi tells how gel derived from fresh aloe vera leaves was air-freighted from Hawaii and applied to the fishermen's burns. The healing of these individuals amazed the medical world.

Bursitis

Bursitis occurs when the fluid in the sacs between bones and tendons (bursae) thickens, becomes resistant, even causes friction when the bones move, and inflammation swells the tissue. Tennis elbow is a well-known example. Bursitis and tendonitis are often confused with one another. While similar, the difference to remember is in the type of pain experienced. Those suffering from tendonitis tend to feel sharp pain upon the start of movement of the afflicted area. The pain associated with bursitis is more of a generalized ache, not as sharp, that increases as movement does.

Recognizing Bursitis

Although bursitis usually occurs in the shoulders and joints, there are more than 140 bursae in the body, including the hips, elbows, knees, and ankles. It is most common among the elderly, but can strike at any age, particularly among athletes and those whose occupations require frequent repetitive movements. Symptoms may include:

- Pain and tenderness
- Redness
- Swelling
- Water retention
- Limited joint motion

What Are the Causes of Bursitis?

- Athletic strain or injury
- Repetitive physical labor
- Overstressed muscles
- Infection
- Calcium deposits in bone sockets
- Food and environmental allergies
- Poor diet
- Poor assimilation of food

What You Can Take

Nutrients

Name	Dosage	Benefits
Vitamin A	10,000 IU daily	Antioxidant and antiinflammatory essential to the formation of collagen.
Vitamin B-complex	100 mg daily	Necessary for maintaining the biochemical balance of all B vitamins when supplementing with any single B vitamin individually.
Vitamin B_{12}	1,000 mcg tablet under the tongue twice daily	Important to the metabolism of nerve tissue.
Vitamin C	500 mg three times daily	Antioxidant and antiinflammatory essential to the formation of collagen.
Bioflavonoid	500 mg of hesperidin, a citrus bioflavonoid, daily	Works with vitamin C in producing and repairing collagen in bursae, and reduces inflammation.
Quercetin	300 mg twice daily	Antioxidant that moderates inflammation and limits injury to bursae.
Zinc	15–30 mg daily	Needed for tissue repair and accelerated healing.

Herbs

Name	Dosage	Benefits
Bromelain	250 mg three times daily	An enzyme derived from pineapple that reduces swelling and promotes healing from injuries.
Turmeric	250 mg capsule between meals	Anti-inflammatory and antihistamine effects.

What You Can Do

✓ Avoid using injured shoulder or other injured bursal area.
✓ Apply ice packs until swelling goes down, then use hot towels to enhance blood circulation and healing.
✓ Test for food and environmental allergies (*see* ALLERGIES).
✓ Avoid sugar and other refined carbohydrates.
✓ Get plenty of rest.
✓ Drink at least 8–10 glasses of pure spring water daily.
✓ Eat plenty of raw fruits and vegetables.
✓ Eat foods high in the following nutrients:
  • Vitamin A, including eggs, milk, cheese, cream, butter, yogurt, salmon, bass, halibut, mackerel, herring, whitefish, sardines, tuna, clams, shrimp, beef, chicken, pistachios, pecans, walnuts, lentils, and soybeans.
  • Vitamin B_{12}, including liver, sardines, mackerel, herring, red snapper, flounder, salmon, lamb, Swiss cheese, blue cheese, eggs, haddock, beef, halibut, anchovies, chicken, turkey, milk, and butter.
  • Vitamin C, including rose hips, acerola cherries, guavas, black currants, red peppers, oranges, grapefruit and other citrus fruits, cabbage, papayas, cantaloupe, and tomatoes.
  • Zinc, including seafood, sardines, oysters, soybeans, soy lecithin, kelp, legumes, meats, liver, eggs, brewer's yeast, mushrooms, poultry, whole grains, and pumpkin and sunflower seeds.

And Try This!
Try drinking a cup of chamomile tea before bed to relieve pain. It will also help you fall asleep!

Did You Know?

Early nutritional research involving bursitis found that daily intramuscular injections of 1,000 mcg of vitamin B_{12} for 7 to 10 days produced relief. Then a follow-up series of 1 or 2 injections per week for 2 to 3 more weeks brought bursitis under control. This regimen developed by Dr. I. S. Klemes, Medical Director of the Ideal Mutual Insurance Company, was described in *The Encyclopedia of Common Diseases* back in 1976. At the time, injecting vitamin B_{12} was the only known way to bypass the intestinal tract, where it is poorly absorbed. Today, taking vitamin B_{12} in tablet form placed under the tongue is recognized as achieving comparable results.

Cancer

Supposedly, we're making gains in the war on cancer. Is the Brooklyn Bridge still on sale for a dollar? When I started practicing medicine, the odds were that 1 in every 5 individuals would develop cancer. Now the odds are 1 in 3. Cancer itself refers to a condition where cells start to reproduce for no apparent reason, resulting in a malignant tumor that often spreads. When left unchecked, such cell reproduction can overwhelm the body's normal defensive systems. There are many different types of cancer (more than 100), depending on where it strikes. Here I will incorporate information on several of the most common, while discussing cancer in general. It is important to note that although some forms are deadlier than others, all are extremely serious and require close medical care. A detailed summary of each is beyond the scope of this book.

Recognizing Cancer

Early warning signs may include the following:

- Bladder cancer: bloody urine, more frequent need to urinate, painful urination
- Breast cancer: lumps in the breast, sore nipples, swelling, redness, and itching
- Colon cancer: bloody stools, chronic diarrhea or constipation
- Cervical and vaginal cancer: bleeding not associated with menstruation, heavier than normal bleeding and/or increased pain during menstruation, unusual discharge

- Prostate cancer: weak urination, lower back pain, and pain in the pelvic region and lower thighs.
- Skin cancer: unusual bumps on or under the skin, including dark, multicolored moles, and sores that bleed or don't heal.

Warning: You *must* see your doctor for further testing at the first sign of concern. Early diagnosis is one of the most important aspects of beating cancer.

What Are the Causes of Cancer?

Identifying all of the potential causes of cancer would require a book (or a shelf full of them) in itself. There are the obvious examples like smoking, environmental pollution, and pesticides we've all heard about. Others you may not be aware of include the following:

- Chlorinated and fluoridated water
- Cured meats, including bacon, beef, ham, hot dogs, and luncheon meats like salami
- Peanuts (due to molds)
- Processed foods that are full of artificial colors, taste-enhancers, preservatives, foaming agents, emulsifiers, and all kinds of other unsafe additives
- Alcohol and drug use
- Caffeine
- Excessive sun exposure
- Lack of exercise
- Stress
- Diet low in fiber
- Diet high in fats
- Diet high in sugar and other refined carbohydrates
- Overweight
- Nutritional deficiencies
- Mercury fillings
- Inherited tendencies

More specific risk factors for individual cancers include:

- Bladder cancer: smoking, caffeine, heavy use of artificial sweeteners, recurring cystitis

- Breast cancer: heavy use of alcohol and/or caffeine, diabetes, diet high in fats, excessive sugar consumption, birth control pills, family history, estrogen therapy
- Cervical and vaginal cancer: sex with many partners, history of venereal disease such as gonorrhea or genital warts, folic acid deficiencies
- Colon cancer: diet low in fiber, chronic constipation, diet high in fats, family history
- Prostate cancer: history of venereal disease, heavy coffee consumption, diet high in fats, repeated prostate infections
- Skin cancer: excessive sun exposure, family history, severe burns

What You Can Take

Nutrients

Name	Dosage	Benefits
Vitamin A (all cancers)	10,000 IU daily. For skin cancer increase dosage to 25,000 IU daily. For cervical and vaginal cancers increase dosage to 60,000 IU daily for two months, then 25,000 IU until Pap smear time—supervised by a medical doctor. *Warning:* Pregnant and pregnancy-eligible women should take no more than 10,000 IU daily.	Important antioxidant and immunity booster, high doses of which are often required by cancer patients.
Vitamin C (all cancers)	500 mg three times daily. For familial polyposis, an inherited condition that leads to colon cancer, take 3,000 mg of time-released vitamin C daily for no less than six months	Well-documented cancer fighter that enhances the immune system.

Name	Dosage	Benefits
Vitamin E (all cancers)	800 IU daily	A strong antioxidant with anti-cancer effects.
Acidophilus (colon cancer)	One capsule containing up to 20 billion units daily	Helps cleanse the colon and keeps waste matter from building up.
Beta-carotene (cervical and vaginal cancer)	25,000 IU daily	Deficiencies linked to cervical dysplasia.
Calcium carbonate (colon cancer)	1,200 mg daily	Can lessen the increase of cancer cells in the colon lining.
Coenzyme Q-10 (breast cancer)	300 mcg daily	Has shown tumor-reducing effects in breast cancer patients.
DHEA (bladder cancer)	100 mg daily *Warning:* Take only under the supervision of a physician. Do not take if you are at risk of hormone-related cancer.	Boosts immune system to resist bladder cancer.
Folic acid (cervical and vaginal cancer)	400 mcg three times daily	Helps prevent and moderate cervical dysplasia.
Kelp (breast cancer)	One tablet daily containing 225 mcg of iodine *Warning:* Higher dosages may be toxic.	High in iodine, deficiencies of which have been linked to breast cancer.
Lycopene (all cancers)	15 mg twice daily	Super antioxidant shown to have remarkable anticancer effects.
Omega-3 (all cancers)	500 mg softgel twice daily	Can prevent or delay the onset of malignancies in many parts of the body.

Name	Dosage	Benefits
Grape seed or pine bark extract (all cancers)	200 mg daily. For colon cancer increase dosage to 1,000 mg daily	Powerful antioxidant that strengthens the immune system.
Quercetin (breast cancer)	500 mg three times daily before meals	Discourages cancer cells from developing.
Resveratrol (skin cancer)	Two 550 mg capsules daily	Has shown promise in the prevention of skin cancer.
Selenium (all cancers)	200 mcg daily	Has strong cancer-preventing effects. Deficiencies have been linked to breast cancer.
Shark cartilage (all cancers)	65 g in powdered form daily or 1 teaspoon in liquid form under the tongue daily	Boosts immunity and can prevent and/or reverse the onset of cancerous tumors.
Shark liver oil, which contains squalene (all cancers)	One or two 570 mg capsules daily	Inhibits cancer-promoting enzymes.
Zinc (all cancers)	15–30 mg daily	Required for proper functioning of cancer-killing immune system T-cells.

Herbs

Name	Dosage	Benefits
Liquid garlic (all cancers)	One teaspoon daily, two teaspoons daily for prostate cancer	Potent all-purpose healer that helps to block the formation of cancer.
Curcumin (skin cancer)	One 300 mg capsule daily	Has shown promise in the prevention of skin cancer.
Ginger (skin cancer)	Two 550 mg capsules daily	May be effective in the prevention of skin cancer.
PC SPES (prostate cancer)	Three 320 mg capsules once or twice daily	Herbal combination that effectively treats prostate cancer and dramatically reduces PSA levels.

What You Can Do

✓ Exercise regularly.
✓ Don't smoke.
✓ Work to relieve stress (*see* STRESS).
✓ Maintain healthy body weight (*see* OVERWEIGHT).
✓ Drink at least 8–10 glasses of pure spring water daily.
✓ Avoid water sources containing chlorine and/or fluoride.
✓ Avoid alcohol, caffeine, all cured meats, peanuts, processed foods, sugar and other refined carbohydrates.
✓ Avoid constipation to prevent colon cancer (*see* CONSTIPATION).
✓ Avoid excessive sun exposure and sunburn to prevent skin cancer. Always apply sunscreen with an SPF of 15 or greater.
✓ Try to minimize your exposure to known environmental carcinogens such as pesticides, air pollution, cleaning solvents, etc.
✓ Speak to a dentist about replacing mercury fillings with those made from safer materials.
✓ Eat organic foods whenever possible.
✓ Eat a pint of acidophilus-rich, unsweetened yogurt daily to discourage colon cancer.
✓ Use extra virgin olive oil in place of butter on whole wheat breads or on salads.
✓ Eat plenty of fresh, raw fruits and vegetables—especially cruciferous vegetables such as broccoli, Brussels sprouts, cabbage, cauliflower, collard greens, kale, and mustard.
✓ Eat tomatoes or tomato-based products high in lycopene more than twice weekly.
✓ Eat foods high in the following nutrients:
   • Vitamin A, including eggs, milk, cheese, cream, butter, yogurt, salmon, bass, halibut, mackerel, herring, whitefish, sardines, tuna, clams, shrimp, beef, chicken, pistachios, pecans, walnuts, lentils, and soybeans.
   • Vitamin C, including rose hips, acerola cherries, guavas, black currants, red peppers, oranges, grapefruit and other citrus fruits, cabbage, papayas, cantaloupe, and tomatoes.
   • Vitamin E, including sunflower seeds, whole wheat, peanuts, cashews, almonds, walnuts, corn oil, soy oil,

soy lecithin, spinach, asparagus, broccoli, oats, and avocados.
- Selenium, including Brazil nuts, fish, organ meats, whole grains, eggs, cabbage, corn, peas, onions, garlic, chicken, beets, barley, and tomatoes.

And Try This!

Try drinking several cups of green tea daily. It is low in caffeine, loaded with antioxidants, and dozens of studies point to its effectiveness in preventing various types of cancer.

Did You Know?

The chemicals in foods and the many that assail us in the environment create free radicals, highly charged molecules that run amuck, attacking other molecules, setting off a chain reaction that injures, changes, or even kills cells. Noted molecular biologist Dr. Bruce Ames of the University of California at Berkeley estimates the number of daily oxidative hits to cellular DNA, the blueprint for cell replication, to be about 10,000 per cell. Many biochemists believe that free radical attacks gradually change the DNA so that it is no longer true to its original instructions, and, over time, create cancerous cells.

Candida Albicans (Yeast) Overgrowth

Even after many decades since *Candida albicans* was first described in medical journals, conventional medicine still scoffs at the idea that there is such a disease. Why? In the intestinal tract or in some other mucus membrane, everybody carries *Candida albicans* yeast—considered harmless—but everybody doesn't manifest the most common symptoms. Because many doctors believe this ailment doesn't exist, patients are not being properly diagnosed. Their symptoms may be treated and basic causes overlooked while the overgrowth of yeast becomes worse.

Recognizing Candida Overgrowth

Candida is four times more common in women than in men. The vast range of candida symptoms stretches their credulity—fifty-one named by the eminent authority Dr. William Crook, author of the best-selling *The Yeast Connection*. Some of the most obvious and generally agreed upon include the following:

* Fatigue, especially after meals
* Vaginal infections
* Vaginal discharge (white and sticky, often accompanied by irritation)
* Frequent and burning urination
* PMS (premenstrual syndrome)
* White patches on the tongue and walls of the mouth
* Intestinal disorders (gas, bloating, cramps, constipation, or chronic diarrhea)
* Headaches
* Migraines
* Mood swings
* Depression
* Inability to concentrate
* Dizziness
* Sleeplessness
* Irritability
* Muscle pain

My system of diagnosing candida is to have cultures taken in the armpits, the anus, under the breasts, the groin, gums, mouth, male genitals, nose, skin lesions, vagina, and vulva. If the yeast is present in many places with a heavy overgrowth, the diagnosis is definitely candida. The second means of diagnosis is a blood test for candida antibodies (called preceptins). Elevated yeast antibodies and a positive test show that the infection is active and threatening.

What Are the Causes of Candida Overgrowth?

- Overuse of antibiotics
- Chemotherapy
- Birth control pills
- Muscle-building steroids
- Diet high in sugar and other refined carbohydrates
- Food allergies
- Alcohol
- Smoking
- Multiple pregnancies
- Weakened immune system
- Underlying serious illness (e.g. AIDS, cancer, diabetes)

What You Can Take

Nutrients

Name	Dosage	Benefits
Vitamin B-complex	100 mg daily	Boosts immunity and aids in proper digestion, both which can be compromised by candida.
Vitamin C (granular)	1 g three times daily in water (a level teaspoon is 1 g), reduce amount if diarrhea occurs	Protects against the many toxins produced by candida.
Multivitamin and mineral complex	As directed on label	A host of nutrients are needed for repair of damage caused by overgrowth of yeast in the body.
Berberine powdered extract	250 mg after all meals	Kills yeast.
Capryllic acid	One to two 1,000 mg capsules twice daily with meals	Kills yeast.
Gamma-linolenic acid (GLA)	Two 500 mg capsules three times daily	Kills yeast.

Name	Dosage	Benefits
Lactobacillus acidophilus	One capsule with 1.5 billion live cells twice daily	Helps replenish friendly bacteria in the colon.

Herbs

Name	Dosage	Benefits
Garlic (odorless)	Two 200 mg capsules daily	Kills yeast.
Olive leaf extract	One 500 mg capsule twice daily for three weeks	Kills yeast.

What You Can Do

✓ Avoid antibiotics, birth control pills, and steroids.
✓ Exercise daily for 30 minutes.
✓ Drink at least 8–10 glasses of pure spring water daily.
✓ Don't smoke.
✓ Test for food and environmental allergies (*see* ALLERGIES).
✓ Test (hair analysis) for toxic levels of mercury and other metals in the body.
✓ Avoid the following foods: all forms of sugar and refined carbohydrates, alcohol, fruit and fruit juice, vinegar, meat and dairy products from cattle treated with antibiotics, aged cheeses, wheat, potatoes, and tomatoes.
✓ Eat more of the following foods: fresh vegetables, fish, free-range poultry, gluten-free grains (brown rice, millet, quinoa), unsweetened yogurt containing live cultures, and cold-pressed oils.

And Try This!

Try drinking several cups of pau d'arco bark tea daily. Pau d'arco bark comes from a Brazilian tree and is known to contain strong antibacterial and antifungal components, good for fighting candida.

Did You Know?

Drugs used to treat candida, most notably Nystatin, can sometimes make the condition worse by causing stronger (drug-resistant) strains of yeast to develop.

Canker Sores

Canker sores, if you've been fortunate enough to avoid them, are ulcers in the mouth, on the cheeks, gums, lips, or tongue. They are shallow red ulcers with a white head that can be as small as the head of a pin or as large as a quarter. They appear singly or in clusters. Just talking, chewing, drinking—especially something hot or cold—or kissing can cause intense pain.

Recognizing Canker Sores

Estimates suggest that as many as 30 percent of Americans suffer from canker sores at some point. They also tend to be more common in women than in men. Symptoms include those noted above, and they generally last anywhere between a few days to nearly a month.

What Are the Causes of Canker Sores?

- Kissing someone who has them
- Nutritional deficiencies (particularly vitamin B_1)
- Food allergies
- Stress
- Fatigue
- Poor dental hygiene
- Poor digestion
- Injury (e.g. biting tongue)

What You Can Take

Nutrients

Name	Dosage	Benefits
Vitamin B-complex	100 mg daily	Prevents and reverses deficiencies in vitamin B_1 that can cause canker sores.
Vitamin C	600 mg combined with 600 mg of bioflavonoids three times daily	Speeds up healing time for canker sores.

Herbs

Name	Dosage	Benefits
Echinacea	300 mg combined with 50 mg of goldenseal root three times daily until sores disappear	Powerful immune system booster proven effective in eliminating canker sores.

What You Can Do

✓ Don't kiss someone with canker sores.
✓ Practice good dental hygiene.
✓ Avoid spicy, salty, or acidic foods.
✓ Avoid processed foods.
✓ Avoid sugar and other refined carbohydrates.
✓ Avoid wheat and citrus fruits.
✓ Avoid coffee and alcohol.
✓ Don't smoke.
✓ Get plenty of rest.
✓ Work to relieve stress (*see* STRESS).
✓ Test for food allergies (*see* ALLERGIES).
✓ Eat raw onions.
✓ Eat foods high in the following nutrients:
  • Vitamin B_1, including brewer's yeast, broccoli, brown rice, Brussels sprouts, eggs, asparagus, fish, poultry, pork, whole grains, legumes, liver, peas, kelp, oatmeals, plums, prunes, raisins, and nuts.

- Vitamin C (not citrus fruits), including rose hips, acerola cherries, guavas, black currants, red peppers, cabbage, papayas, cantaloupe, and tomatoes.

And Try This!

Try drinking normal-strength yarrow tea. It has been found to be an effective mouthwash for canker sores, and was allegedly a favorite wound herb of the warrior Achilles.

Did You Know?

For decades many biochemists knew that a deficiency of B-complex vitamins could cause canker sores to erupt. An Israeli study had shown that 28.2 percent of individuals who develop them frequently lack sufficient B vitamins. However, they didn't know which specific member of the B-complex family was most deficient. Then biochemists in Tel Aviv researched the problem for over a year and found that 70 percent of patients with recurrent canker sores were deficient in vitamin B_1, compared with just 4 percent in the control group.

Cardiomyopathy

Cardiomyopathy refers to any set of conditions that impair the heart's ability to pump blood, a common cause of congestive heart failure. Up until recently modern medicine has provided cardiomyopathy patients with two bad alternatives: a heart transplant, with its frightening risks, or death. But prospects are actually far brighter than these narrow mainstream alternatives indicate, thanks to the pioneering research of Dr. Peter H. Langsjoen, of the Scott and White Clinic in Temple, Texas, involving coenzyme Q-10 and its importance in treating and preventing cardiovascular disease.

Recognizing Cardiomyopathy

- Reduced ability of heart to contract
- Poor pumping of blood
- Fluid in lungs
- Shortness of breath

What Are the Causes of Cardiomyopathy?

- Heredity
- Deficiency of vitamin B_1
- Deficiency of zinc and copper
- Low thyroid function
- Poor metabolism
- Toxicity
- Viral infection
- Weak heart muscle

What You Can Take

Nutrients

Name	Dosage	Benefits
Vitamin B-complex	100 mg daily	Assures balanced intake of all B vitamins.
Vitamin B_1	100 mg daily	Helps to assure strong thrust of the heart.
Coenzyme Q-10	100 mg daily continuously	Strengthens heart muscle and energy.
L-carnitine	500 mg three times daily	Increases heart's ability to use available energy, and lengthens time patient can exercise.
Taurine	500 mg three times daily	Helps heart energy, thrust and ability to beat with regularity.
Copper	2 mg daily	Teams with zinc to assure a strong heartbeat.
Magnesium	200 to 400 mg three times daily *Warning:* Kidney patients should not take supplemental magnesium without a doctor's close monitoring.	Helps strengthen and regularize heartbeat in cardiomyopathy.

Zinc	30 mg daily	Aids heart pumping vigor and helps to relieve shortness of breath.

Herbs

Name	Dosage	Benefits
Hawthorn	300 mg twice daily	Increases energy for heart, improves pumping ability and dilates arteries.

What You Can Do

✓ Eat foods that are high in the following nutrients:
- Vitamin B₁, including sesame seeds, Brazil nuts, pecans, millet, buckwheat, oats, whole wheat, lentils, brown rice, egg yolks, salmon, wheat germ, blackstrap molasses, and supplements.
- Coenzyme Q-10, including mackerel, salmon, sardines, and spinach.
- Carnitine, including flesh meat, liver, and poultry.
- Taurine, found in meat.
- Copper, including mushrooms, liver, wheat germ, blackstrap molasses, hazelnuts, walnuts, salmon, cashews, and ginseng.
- Magnesium, including blackstrap molasses, sunflower seeds, wheat germ, almonds, soy lecithin, pecans, oats, brown rice, barley, salmon, corn, avocados, and bananas.
- Zinc, including herring, wheat germ, sesame seeds, blackstrap molasses, liver, soybeans, sunflower seeds, egg yolk, chicken, brewer's yeast, oats, and whole wheat.

✓ Increase exercise gradually as condition improves and as specified and monitored by your doctor.

And Try This!
By proceeding with faith in your treatment, you will avoid worry, which tends to make nutrients less available and arteries more constricted, delaying healing.

Did You Know?

Centuries before England's Dr. William Harvey's discovery—in the early 1600s—that the heart's function is to pump blood throughout the body, people took various forms of the herb hawthorn to allay chest pains caused by various heart ailments including what is now known as cardiomyopathy.

Carpal Tunnel Syndrome

It seems that meat cutters, professional pianists, tailors, production line assemblers, seamstresses, supermarket checkers, carpenters, and computer operators would have little in common. Not true. They make innumerable repetitious movements with their hands and wrists, and they are among occupational and artistic groups most likely to suffer from carpal tunnel syndrome (CTS), a modern ailment afflicting millions. And (whether they know it or not) they should also share hope—there's light at the end of the carpal tunnel!

Recognizing Carpal Tunnel Syndrome

- Numbness, tingling and pain in the fingers (especially the thumb and first three fingers), hands, or wrists
- Often disabling, the pain may be accompanied by weakness of the hands and an inability to grasp and lift even light objects
- Waking up with fingers curled and stiff

What Are the Causes of Carpal Tunnel Syndrome?

CTS is one of the more severe forms of what are called Repetitive Strain Injuries. The major cause of CTS involves crowded quarters in the carpus, eight small bones that form a tunnel in the wrist. Going through that tunnel are two important body parts: a ligament that joins the two forearm bones at their ends a few inches from where the palm begins, and near it, the median nerve that travels the long distance from the hand up to the neck. Under certain conditions, much repeated action causes the ligament to swell until it presses on the sensitive nerve, causing CTS. Contributing factors can include:

- Repetitious movements with hands and wrists
- Lack of vitamin B$_6$
- Bad posture
- Pregnancy (water retention)
- Menopause
- Diabetes
- Arthritis
- Low thyroid function
- Overweight
- Nerve disorders

What You Can Take

Nutrients

Name	Dosage	Benefits
Vitamin B$_6$	100-200 mg daily *Warning:* Pregnant women should consult with their obstetrician before taking a higher amount.	Studies point to dramatic improvements in correcting CTS.

What You Can Do

✓ Be hesitant about agreeing to surgery.
✓ Avoid salt and salty foods (they promote water retention).
✓ Avoid processed foods.
✓ Avoid alcohol, barbiturates, cortisone, and birth control pills.
✓ Keep feet on floor to maintain knees and hips at a 90-degree angle while at a computer.
✓ Wear lightweight splints during the night to support wrists.

✓ Maintain a healthy body weight (*see* OVERWEIGHT).
✓ Test for low thyroid function (*see* HYPOTHYROIDISM).
✓ Eat foods high in vitamin B$_6$, including brewer's yeast, brown rice, whole wheat, royal jelly, soybeans, rye, lentils, sunflower seeds, alfalfa, salmon, wheat germ, tuna, bran, walnuts, cashews, peanuts, peas, liver, avocados, beans, turkey, oats, chicken, halibut, lamb, and bananas.

And Try This!

Try taking frequent breaks when engaged in repetitive tasks (like typing), and stretching or shaking out your hands and fingers whenever possible.

Did You Know?

Dr. John Ellis, the world's foremost expert on CTS, and his colleague Dr. Karl Folkes conducted a double-blind study demonstrating that CTS sufferers are invariably deficient in vitamin B$_6$ and overcome this condition when receiving proper supplementation. In several instances, patients who had endured CTS for as long as 8 years recovered completely following treatment with vitamin B$_6$.

Cataracts

Cataracts are a clouding or opacity of the eye lenses, impairing or totally blocking vision. A serious condition that affects millions, they occur most among the elderly, and are also the world's leading cause of blindness. Surgery is the standard conventional approach to treating cataracts, but results are often mixed.

Recognizing Cataracts

Cataracts are best characterized as a steady, usually pain-free loss of vision. Frequent eye exams are the best way to detect the condition, particularly as you get older.

What Are the Causes of Cataracts?

Cataracts are caused by free radicals, highly reactive oxygen molecules, attacking proteins in the lenses of the eyes, which creates clouding. Contributing include:

- Aging
- Smoking
- Diabetes
- Excessive sun exposure

What You Can Take

Nutrients

Name	Dosage	Benefits
Vitamin A	10,000 IU daily	Improves night vision.
Vitamin B-complex	100 mg daily	Essential for metabolism of nutrients in the eyes.
Vitamin C	500 mg three times daily	Prevents cataract formation.
Vitamin E	400 IU daily	Antioxidant that protects and activates glutathione.
Cysteine	200 mg daily	Replenishes glutathione, richly present in healthy lenses and deficient in those with cataracts.
Glutamic acid	200 mg daily	Replenishes glutathione, richly present in healthy lenses and deficient in those with cataracts.
Glycine	200 mg daily	Replenishes glutathione, richly present in healthy lenses and deficient in those with cataracts.
Selenium	200 mcg daily	Protects against deficiencies common among cataract patients.

Herbs

Name	Dosage	Benefits
Bilberry extract	40–60 mg two to three times daily	Prevents hemorrhages, increases blood circulation, and strengthens connective tissue in the eyes.

What You Can Do

✓ Have regular eye exams, particularly as you get older.
✓ Avoid excessive sun exposure (wear sunglasses that protect against UVA).
✓ Don't smoke.
✓ Avoid alcohol and caffeine.
✓ Avoid milk, sugar, and other refined carbohydrates.
✓ Drink at least 8–10 glasses of pure spring water daily.
✓ Eat plenty of fresh fruits and vegetables (especially spinach).
✓ Eat foods high in vitamin A, including eggs, yogurt, salmon, bass, halibut, mackerel, herring, whitefish, sardines, tuna, clams, shrimp, beef, chicken, pistachios, pecans, walnuts, lentils, and soybeans.
✓ Eat foods high in vitamin C, including rose hips, acerola cherries, guavas, black currants, red peppers, oranges, grapefruit and other citrus fruits, cabbage, papayas, cantaloupe, and tomatoes.
✓ Eat foods high in vitamin E, including sunflower seeds, whole wheat, peanuts, cashews, almonds, walnuts, corn oil, soy oil, soy lecithin, spinach, asparagus, broccoli, butter, oats, and avocados.
✓ Eat foods high in selenium, including Brazil nuts, fish, organ meats, whole grains, eggs, cabbage, corn, peas, onions, garlic, chicken, beets, barley, and tomatoes.

And Try This!
Depend on vitamin C supplements, as indicated, rather than foods rich in this vitamin. Strangely, studies show that only vitamin C supplements are effective in cataract prevention and control.

Did You Know?

During World War II, pilots in Britain's Royal Air Force found their night vision was much keener after eating bilberry preserves, and so bilberry became a regular part of their night missions. Research that followed proved bilberry helps the eyes in other important ways, too—in cataract prevention, in macular degeneration, and possibly, even in glaucoma.

Cavities

So you think that brushing your teeth twice daily, flossing them regularly, going easy on sweets, and having a dental checkup and cleaning every six months are going to keep you from having cavities? Think again! They provide a great deal of protection, but not all. A study by Dr. William Howard, of the University of Oregon School of Dentistry, shows that stress of all kinds causes teeth to develop cavities in two ways: by changing the balance of microorganisms in the mouth in favor of harmful bacteria over friendly, and through stealing minerals and other nutrients from bones and teeth.

Recognizing Cavities

See your dentist. Short of a toothache, it's difficult to detect cavities without regular dental examinations.

What Are the Causes of Cavities?

- Poor oral hygiene
- Diet high in sugar and other refined carbohydrates (especially white flour)
- Nutritional deficiencies
- Stress
- Family history

What You Can Take

Nutrients

Name	Dosage	Benefits
Vitamin B-complex	100 mg daily	Important for maintaining healthy gums.
Vitamin C	500 mg three times daily	Protects against inflammation and bacterial infection in the mouth.
Multimineral complex	As directed on label	Contains every nutrient required for healthy teeth and bones.

What You Can Do

✓ Brush, gargle, and floss as soon as possible after eating.
✓ Schedule two checkups a year with your dentist.
✓ Avoid sugar and other refined carbohydrates (especially white flour).
✓ Avoid soft drinks.
✓ Work to relieve stress (*see* STRESS).
✓ Choose snacks that don't stick to your teeth such as nuts, meats, olives, cheese, and yogurt.
✓ Eat plenty of fresh fruits and vegetables.
✓ Eat foods high in vitamin C, including rose hips, acerola cherries, guavas, black currants, red peppers, oranges, grapefruit and other citrus fruits, cabbage, papayas, cantaloupe, and tomatoes.

And Try This!

When you're away from home and can't brush or floss your teeth after eating cavity-producing foods, try doing the next best thing: Take a mouthful of water and swish it around for 10 to 15 seconds. This will loosen food particles that you can spit out.

Did You Know?

Fluoride added to city water to protect children against cavities is of dubious value and can cause harm, as many surveys have indicated. Dr. Stephen Moss, professor and chairman of Pediatric Dentistry at New York University College of Dentistry, claims that if there have been improvements in children's teeth, this is due to the heightened awareness of parents in starting early to prevent cavities in their children through better dental hygiene and nutrition.

Celiac Disease

Adults, take note! It is common to think of celiac disease (gluten intolerance) as a disorder of infants and small children. Several decades ago this was true. However, now more and more adults are victimized by celiac disease, also known as gluten enteropathy, idiopathic steatorrhea, or nontropical sprue.

Recognizing Celiac Disease

Celiac disease can strike at any age, especially in children during the first year of life. Doctors often fail to properly diagnose it, a mistake that can result in serious consequences such as the eventual development of autoimmune diseases like diabetes, lupus, thyroid disorders, and arthritis. Early symptoms of celiac disease may include the following:

- Diarrhea
- Gas
- Bloating
- Nausea
- Vomiting
- Eczema
- Foul stools
- Fatigue
- Depression
- Irritability
- Weight loss
- Cramps
- Joint and/or bone pain
- Anemia
- Food and environmental allergies

What Are the Causes of Celiac Disease?

In susceptible people, allergy to gluten causes inflammation of delicate intestinal membranes and destruction of their villi, tiny hairlike projections that absorb nutrients. Once they're gone, they can't grow back. This can lead to destruction of the stomach lining, as well as the intestinal lining—making the absorption of nutrients all the more difficult (especially fats and fat-soluble vitamins), which will eventually lead to nutritional deficiencies.

What You Can Take

Nutrients (For Children)

Name	Dosage	Benefits
Vitamin B-complex	50 mg daily	Necessary for maintaining the biochemical balance of all B vitamins when supplementing with any single B vitamin individually.
Vitamin B$_6$	50 mg daily	Required for proper digestion.

Nutrients (For Adults)

Name	Dosage	Benefits
Vitamin B-complex	100 mg daily	Necessary for maintaining the biochemical balance of all B vitamins when supplementing with any single B vitamin individually.
Vitamin B$_6$	100 mg daily	Required for proper digestion.
Vitamin D	400 IU capsule daily or a tablespoon of cod liver oil	Celiac disease is indirectly related to vitamin D deficiency.
Folic acid	400–800 mcg daily	Folic acid deficiency is often associated with celiac disease.

What You Can Do

✓ Eliminate gluten-containing wheat, barley, rye, and oats from the diet.

✓ Read labels carefully for gluten, as it is a common ingredient in packaged foods such as soy sauce, salad dressings, ketchup, mustard, hot dogs, cold cuts, sausages, baked beans, white vinegar, some soups, and even "nutritional supplements."

✓ Gluten may also appear on labels under the following names: hydrolyzed vegetable protein, texturized vegetable protein, hydrolyzed plant protein, malt, modified food starch, and natural flavorings.

✓ Avoid dairy products.

✓ Avoid sugar and other forms of refined carbohydrates.

✓ Avoid alcohol.

✓ Add 4 ounces of broiled liver to your diet three times a week.

✓ Eat foods high in vitamin B_6, including brewer's yeast, brown rice, whole wheat, royal jelly, soybeans, rye, lentils, sunflower seeds, alfalfa, salmon, wheat germ, tuna, bran, walnuts, cashews, peanuts, peas, liver, avocados, beans, turkey, oats, chicken, halibut, lamb, and bananas.

✓ Eat foods high in vitamin D, including cod liver oil, eggs, herring, organ meats, salmon, and sardines.

✓ Eat foods high in folic acid, including whole grains, wheat germ, bran, brown rice, liver, beef, barley, chicken, tuna, salmon, lentils, legumes, brewer's yeast, oranges, mushrooms, and green leafy vegetables.

And Try This!

Try shopping at your local health food store for gluten-free foods such as pasta, cereals, and baked goods. You'll be surprised by the variety of tasty options!

Did You Know?

The late Carlton Fredericks, an outstanding nutritionist, once told me that Greek schizophrenics and paranoids improved markedly during the World War II Nazi occupation when bread, a staple in the Greek diet, became scarce. Based on what happened in Greece, a New York psychiatrist cut wheat out of the diets of hospitalized schizophrenics and slashed the length of their hospitalization compared with those who continued eating wheat products.

Cellulite

As a woman, Mother Nature should be somewhat embarrassed that she designed the skin of females so that it is far more prone than that of men to develop cellulite: lumpy fat deposits on the thighs, buttocks, and upper arms. Prevent this lumpiness, pitting, and dimpling and you won't have to join the Cellulite Set. If you're already a member, there's still hope. However, you need to know more about your skin and best ways of coping with cellulite.

Recognizing Cellulite

You've recognized it all right—or you wouldn't have turned to this section!

What Are the Causes of Cellulite?

Although cellulite is visible in the skin (epidermis), the trouble starts below that in the dermis. A woman's dermis is half as thick as that of a man's and thins even more with age. One level deeper (in the upper part of the subcutaneous layer) women have cells called fat chambers, separated by arching and radial connective tissue handcuffed to connective tissue of the dermis. Fat cells of men are far smaller and are held in place and shape by a network of restraining connective tissue. As the dermis in women thins and loosens with age, the containing connective tissue also thins and becomes flabby. Then opportunistic fat cells below enlarge and push up into the also thinning dermis. Factors that contribute to the process include:

- Lack of exercise
- Overeating
- Poor circulation

What You Can Take

Nutrients

Name	Dosage	Benefits
Vitamin C	500 mg three times daily	Keeps collagen strong. Collagen helps make connective tissue better able to restrain fat cells from expanding and migrating upward and becoming visible cellulite lumps.

Herbs

Name	Dosage	Benefits
Centella asiatica	30 mg after each meal	Helps to balance and normalize the metabolism in connective tissue.

What You Can Do

✓ Walk briskly for 30 minutes 4 or 5 days weekly.
✓ Enlist another person with cellulite to walk with you so that you're more likely to stick to your schedule.
✓ If you find walking a bore, add competitive sports to your routine such as tennis, golf, or volleyball.
✓ Drink at least 8–10 glasses of pure spring water daily.
✓ Follow a low-fat, high-fiber diet rich in complex carbohydrates and fresh fruits and vegetables.
✓ Eat foods high in vitamin C, including rose hips, acerola cherries, guavas, black currants, red peppers, oranges, grapefruit and other citrus fruits, cabbage, papayas, cantaloupe, and tomatoes.

And Try This!

Try slowly massaging cellulite lumps with a loofah and almond scrub (available in most health food stores). This improves blood circulation, which helps to diminish cellulite.

Did You Know?

It's true that too little exercise and too much food invite cellulite. However, don't exercise too strenuously and crash diet to lose weight too quickly. Such diets are deficient in nutrients and harmful. Further, if you're middle-aged, overweight, and under-exercising, your connective tissue already may show deterioration. Undernutrition weakens it faster, and cellulite lumps show even more than before.

Circulatory Disorders

That big pump within the left side of your chest is doing its best to thrust oxygenated, nutrient-laden blood to each of your trillions of cells to keep you healthy and young. But if the flow of blood is impaired because of a circulatory disorder, there can be severe damage, especially if it isn't recognized and treated early.

Circulatory disorders can appear in several forms. For instance, in arteriosclerosis, calcium deposits form along the artery walls, causing them to thicken and harden. In the case of atherosclerosis, there is a buildup of fatty substances along the artery walls. Both conditions have the same effect on circulation: hypertension, or high blood pressure, where the blood exerts greater force against the walls of the narrowed and more rigid blood vessels. This can lead to such dangerous consequences as stroke, angina pectoris (chest pain), kidney damage, and heart attacks. Other circulatory problems can lead to gangrene and limb amputations.

Recognizing Circulatory Disorders

Circulatory disorders are difficult to diagnose on your own and need to be properly tested for by a physician. However, symptoms suggestive of blood flow problems can include the following:

- Restricted sense of feeling, tingling, or intermittent numbness in extremities
- Loss of normal color or onset of bluish color in extremities
- High blood pressure (hypertension)
- Ulcerous feet
- Gangrene

What Are the Causes of Circulatory Disorders?

- Family history
- Smoking
- Stress
- Lack of exercise
- Overweight
- Varicose veins
- Diabetes
- Blocking arterial plaque
- Nutritional deficiencies (especially vitamin C)
- Toxic levels of heavy metals such as lead and mercury in the body

What You Can Take

Nutrients

Name	Dosage	Benefits
Vitamin B-complex	50–100 mg daily	Necessary for maintaining the biochemical balance of all B vitamins when supplementing with any single B vitamin individually.
Vitamin B_6	250 mg daily	Enhances blood circulation.

Name	Dosage	Benefits
Vitamin C	500–1,000 mg three times daily	Prevents buildup of harmful plaque in the arteries and promotes healing in already damaged arteries.
Vitamin E	400–1,200 IU daily	Powerful antioxidant that attacks harmful (LDL) cholesterol and prevents clogged arteries.
Chondroitin sulphate	400 mg three times daily	Effectively thins blood, reduces blood fats, and helps maintain smooth and elastic arteries.
Folic acid	5 mg daily	Reduces levels of homocysteine in the blood, a prime risk factor for heart attacks.
Lycopene	15 mg twice daily	Super antioxidant that prevents harmful (LDL) cholesterol from oxidizing and forming plaque that restricts blood flow.
Omega-3 fatty acids	1,000 mg softgel twice daily	Helps raise good (HDL) cholesterol, lowers triglycerides, and lessens chance of heart attack.

Herbs

Name	Dosage	Benefits
Garlic (odorless)	1 teaspoon three times daily	Lowers blood pressure and helps prevent abnormal blood clotting.
Gugulipid	25 mg gugulsterones three times daily	Reduces risk of heart attack, helps lower cholesterol and triglycerides.

What You Can Do

✓ Don't smoke.
✓ Avoid caffeine.

✓ Avoid sugar and other refined carbohydrates.

✓ Work to relieve stress (*see* STRESS).

✓ Exercise for 30 minutes four to five times per week.

✓ Drink at least 8–10 glasses of pure spring water daily.

✓ Maintain healthy body weight (*see* OVERWEIGHT).

✓ Consume a diet high in fiber to lower cholesterol levels.

✓ Test (hair analysis) for toxic levels of heavy metals such as lead and mercury in the body.

✓ Eat fresh fruit and vegetables (part of the successful circulation improvement program of Dr. Dean Ornish).

✓ Eat foods high in vitamin B$_6$, including brewer's yeast, brown rice, whole wheat, royal jelly, soybeans, rye, lentils, sunflower seeds, alfalfa, salmon, wheat germ, tuna, bran, walnuts, cashews, peanuts, peas, liver, avocados, beans, turkey, oats, chicken, halibut, lamb, and bananas.

✓ Eat foods high in folic acid, including whole grains, oats, whole wheat, wheat germ, bran, brown rice, liver, milk, beef, barley, chicken, tuna, salmon, lentils, legumes, brewer's yeast, cheese, oranges, asparagus, mushrooms, and green leafy vegetables.

✓ Eat foods high in vitamin B$_{12}$, including liver, sardines, mackerel, herring, red snapper, salmon, Swiss cheese, eggs, beef, and halibut.

✓ Eat foods high in vitamin C, including rose hips, acerola cherries, guavas, black currants, red peppers, oranges, grapefruit and other citrus fruits, cabbage, papayas, cantaloupe, and tomatoes.

✓ Eat foods high in vitamin E, including sunflower seeds, whole wheat, peanuts, cashews, almonds, walnuts, olive oil, corn oil, soy oil, soy lecithin, spinach, asparagus, broccoli, butter oats, and avocados.

And Try This!

Try chelation therapy, a safe and effective means of ridding your arteries of circulation-impeding plaque as well as toxic heavy metals such as lead and mercury. Chelation can be done orally, as well as intravenously. Your health food store can direct you to physicians trained in chelation therapy.

Did You Know?

Stress can sabotage your arteries, as demonstrated by a study of 26 patients with chest pains symptomatic of coronary heart disease by Alan C. Yeung, M.D., of Harvard Medical School. Before the test, the intima—inside of their coronary arteries—were found to be "relatively smooth," irregular (somewhat plaqued) and "stenosed," almost plaque-clogged.

Stress caused the stenosed arteries to constrict by 24 percent. Arteries with little plaque constricted by 9 percent. However, smooth and healthy arteries stayed the same or even expanded.

Colds and Flu

One of the great curses of the human race is the common cold. In fact, most folks come down with several a year. Many different viruses (hundreds!) cause colds, including the flu virus, which is why they sometimes get confused. Both are highly contagious viral infections of the upper respiratory tract, but their symptoms are different.

Recognizing a Cold

- Slow onset
- Not always accompanied by fever
- Sneezing and runny nose
- Watery eyes
- Clogged breathing
- Chest discomfort accompanied by wheezing
- Headaches
- Sore or burning throat
- Hoarseness

Recognizing the Flu

- Swift and overwhelming onset
- High fever
- Weakening of entire body
- Aches and pains throughout the body
- Chills
- Extreme fatigue
- Sore throat
- Burning sensation in chest
- Dry hacking cough
- Severe headaches
- Aches around and behind the eyes

What Are the Causes of Colds and Flu?

Exposure to someone else suffering from the cold or flu is the primary cause of both conditions. However, even though colds and flu are highly contagious, becoming infected is not merely a matter of getting exposed. Nor is it true that being physically cold causes colds. The reason some of us seem to catch every bug going around—including colds and flu—is a weakened immune system. Contributing factors can include the following:

- Fatigue
- Stress
- Allergies of the nose and throat
- A diet high in sugar and other refined carbohydrates
- Nutritional deficiencies

What You Can Take

Nutrients

Name	Dosage	Benefits
Vitamin A	10,000 IU daily	Protects mucus membranes and fights infections.
Vitamin B-complex	100 mg daily	Necessary for maintaining the biochemical balance of all B vitamins when supplementing with any single B vitamin.

Name	Dosage	Benefits
Vitamin B_5	300–1,000 mg daily	Stimulates and strengthens the immune system.
Vitamin C	1,000–8,000 mg daily	Super immune booster that directly attacks cold and flu viruses, and reduces the severity and duration of cold symptoms.
Gamma linolenic acid (GLA)	500 mg capsule daily	Anti-inflammatory effects. Relieves fever and muscle soreness associated with flu.
Omega-3 essential fatty acids: EPA and DHA	1,000 mg softgel daily	Helpful for people who are prone to frequent colds.
Zinc	2 zinc lozenges at start of cold, then 1 lozenge every three hours for no more than three days (add 2 mg of copper daily if taken beyond that time)	Essential for strong immune system. Defends against many viruses that cause colds and reduces duration and severity of colds.

Herbs

Name	Dosage	Benefits
Astragalus	400 mg twice daily	Reduces frequency of cold and flu by boosting immune system.
Echinacea and goldenseal (combined in single supplement)	500 mg tablet containing 300 mg of echinacea, 50 mg of goldenseal, and 150 mg of additional herbs	Boosts immune system and can fight off a cold before it starts if taken at the first sign of cold symptoms.
Garlic (odorless)	400 mg four times daily	Reduces severity and duration of colds and flu.
Andrographis paniculata	300 mg four times daily	Reduces cold and flu symptoms and strengthens the immune system.

What You Can Do

- ✓ Practice good hygiene: Wash hands frequently, and don't put fingers in mouth or eyes.
- ✓ Limit exposure to others infected with cold and flu.
- ✓ Drink at least 8–10 glasses of pure spring water daily.
- ✓ Get plenty of rest.
- ✓ Don't smoke.
- ✓ Avoid alcohol and drugs.
- ✓ Avoid sugar and other refined carbohydrates.
- ✓ Work to relieve stress (*see* STRESS).
- ✓ Dab powdered vitamin C (in the form of sodium ascorbate) in the nostrils using a pinch on your fingertip.
- ✓ Eat foods high in vitamin A, including eggs, milk, cheese, cream, butter, yogurt, salmon, bass, halibut, mackerel, herring, whitefish, sardines, tuna, clams, shrimp, beef, chicken, pistachios, pecans, walnuts, lentils, and soybeans.
- ✓ Eat foods high in vitamin C, including rose hips, acerola cherries, guavas, black currants, red peppers, oranges, grapefruit and other citrus fruits, cabbage, papayas, cantaloupe, and tomatoes.
- ✓ Eat foods high in zinc, including seafood, sardines, oysters, soybeans, soy lecithin, kelp, legumes, meats, liver, eggs, brewer's yeast, mushrooms, poultry, whole grains, and pumpkin and sunflower seeds.
- ✓ Don't forget the chicken soup: it opens nasal passages and helps get rid of colds.

And Try This!

Try breathing warm air over a basin of hot water, using a bath towel over your head. It helps to relieve nasal congestion and speeds up healing.

Did You Know?

Nancy Beckham reports an unusual story in her *Family Guide to Natural Remedies*. In a 10-year study, Norwegian lumberjacks accidentally found a way of preventing colds while using vitamin C powder for another purpose. The pot-belly stoves in their mountain cabins burned pine wood and gave off toxic substances that irritated their nasal mucus membranes, turning them red, so they wisely dabbed powdered vitamin C (sodium ascorbate) on them. This form of vitamin C doesn't sting in the nostrils like plain ascorbic acid powder. The lumberjacks accomplished more than just conquering nasal irritation, writes Beckham. They didn't catch a cold in all their time in the mountains. However, things changed when they returned to their valley homes.

Congestive Heart Failure

A condition of this kind is so serious that patients should always get approval of their doctor for any nutrition or exercise regimen that they wish to adopt to deal with it.

Recognizing Congestive Heart Failure

Symptoms:

- Overwhelming fatigue
- Trouble in breathing while lying down
- Shortness of breath
- Fluid accumulation in the lungs
- Swollen ankles and feet
- Enlarged heart
- Limited ability to exercise

What Are the Causes of Congestive Heart Failure?

The heart can't pump blood as fast and forcefully as needed, a condition that can be caused by many other ailments, as follows:

- Anemia
- High blood pressure
- Hyperthyroidism
- Heart arrhythmias (irregular beating)
- Heart attacks
- Nutritional deficiencies

What You Can Take

Nutrients

Name	Dosage	Benefits
Arginine	5–10 g daily	A major ingredient for nitric oxide that increases blood flow.
L-carnitine	500 mg two times daily	Improves ability to exercise after being taken for six months.
Taurine	500 mg three times daily	Strengthens the heart's ability to pump.
Magnesium	400 mg daily	Compensates for loss of this mineral in CHF.

Herbs

Name	Dosage	Benefits
Hawthorn	50 to 300 mg two times daily	Increases the heart's ability to contract; helps blood reach the extremities; protects heart tissue from damage by oxidation.

What You Can Do

✓ Eat fresh fruits and vegetables.
✓ Be checked by your doctor for anemia.
✓ Be checked for blood levels of magnesium.
✓ Start a mild exercise program only if approved and monitored by your doctor.
✓ Include some meat in your diet. This contains carnitine.

And Try This!

Ask your doctor if 50 mg of vitamin B-complex daily can help your condition. Low blood and blood plasma levels of vitamin B_1 were discovered in 30 consecutive heart failure outpatients in a Tampa, Florida clinic.

Did You Know?

Alternative doctors specializing in cardiovascular ailments find that many patients give up too early on supplements. Improvement sometimes takes months or even a year to show, particularly when taking coenzyme Q-10. Further, CHF patients should not abruptly stop taking coenzyme Q-10, because there could be danger of a relapse.

Constipation

It doesn't seem fair! You take a lot of antacids for excess stomach acid, and you develop constipation. You take painkillers, antidepressants, antihypertensives, or diuretics regularly, and the same thing happens. Add natural causes for too few, irregular, or painful bowel movements—plus impacted and hard fecal matter—and you wonder how it's even possible to be a "regular" guy or gal.

Recognizing Constipation

Experts differ on just how many bowel movements should be considered healthy, but most agree on at least one per day. Two or three is ideal. Stools should be soft and float in the toilet bowl. Hard stools that sink are a sign of constipation.

In addition to infrequent bowel movements, constipation is often accompanied by a number of related symptoms. These can include:

- Depression
- Irritability
- Gas
- Hemorrhoids
- Diverticulitis
- Indigestion
- Insomnia
- Fatigue
- Stomach cramps
- Body odor
- Obesity

What Are the Causes of Constipation?

- Drinking too little water
- Lack of fiber in the diet
- Diet too high in protein and/or fat
- Highly processed foods
- Food allergies
- Low thyroid function
- Nutritional deficiencies (especially folic acid)
- Pregnancy
- Lack of exercise
- Overuse of laxatives
- Yeast overgrowth
- Drug reactions

What You Can Take

Nutrients

Name	Dosage	Benefits
Vitamin C	2,000 mg daily and above to bowel tolerance (onset of diarrhea)	Establishing a level just prior to the onset of diarrhea can increase regularity.
Calcium	1,000 mg daily and related magnesium at 250 mg daily	Improper balance between calcium and magnesium intake can produce constipation.
Folic acid	600–1,200 mcg daily	Deficiency of folic acid is almost always related to constipation.

Herbs

Name	Dosage	Benefits
Cascara sagrada	Two to five capsules daily	Best-researched herb for treating constipation.

What You Can Do

✓ Drink at least 8–10 glasses of pure spring water daily.
✓ Get daily exercise: bending exercises like touching the floor or lying on your back and drawing your knees up to your chest help move the bowels.
✓ Test for low thyroid function (*see* HYPOTHYROIDISM).
✓ Test for food allergies (*see* ALLERGIES).

✓ Include whole grain breads and cereals for breakfast.

✓ Eat 1 pint of plain, cultured yogurt daily to implant friendly bacteria in the colon.

✓ Avoid laxatives, opting for natural alternatives instead such as 3–4 dried apricots, a saucer of sauerkraut, a glass of sauerkraut juice, a saucer of cooked prunes, or warm prune juice.

✓ Increase consumption of the following foods: fresh fruits and vegetables (especially apples, carrots, bananas, and cabbage), dried fruits, oat bran, brown rice, psyllium seeds, flaxseeds and flaxseed oil, beans, and garlic.

✓ Avoid the following foods: fried foods, sugar and other refined carbohydrates (especially white flour), dairy products (except yogurt), soft drinks, coffee, and alcohol.

And Try This!

Try taking the homeopathic remedy Nat mur at a dosage of 6x three times daily. It can be especially helpful for constipation patients suffering from stubborn stool retention.

Did You Know?

In *Health Survival in the 21st Century,* Ross Horne states that the transit time for the typical Western diet is roughly 72 hours, compared with 24 hours elsewhere, giving potent toxins ample time to be absorbed in the body by way of bile circulation and to set up the irritation that leads to appendicitis and colon cancer.

Cramps

Ouch! And sleep was supposed to be a time to *relax*. Nothing can wake you up faster than a late-night cramp. Instant agony! But thankfully, there's a lot you can do to make sure the only thing you have to fear about dozing off is the sound of that nasty alarm clock in the morning.

Recognizing Cramps

Other than those associated with exercise, cramps mainly occur at night. They tend to affect the legs more than other parts of the body and commonly turn the calf muscles into wickedly painful knots.

What Are the Causes of Cramps?

- Nutritional deficiencies (especially calcium and vitamin E)
- Exercising too hard or without adequate warm-up
- Dehydration
- Bending in a different than usual way
- Standing or squatting for a long period of time
- Heavier lifting than usual
- Sleeping with a leg twisted
- Smoking
- Poor circulation
- Crash dieting
- Anemia

What You Can Take

Nutrients

Name	Dosage	Benefits
Vitamin C	500 mg three times daily	Improves circulation.
Vitamin D	400 IU daily	Essential to the absorption of calcium.
Vitamin E	400 IU daily	Prevents leg cramps at night.
Calcium	800–1,000 mg daily	Key mineral in the transmission of signals throughout nervous system.
Magnesium	500 mg daily	Enables muscles to relax.
Potassium	500 mg daily	Helps normalize muscles.

What You Can Do

✓ Always warm up before vigorous exercise.
✓ Avoid crash diets.
✓ Don't smoke.
✓ Drink at least 8–10 glasses of pure spring water daily.
✓ Add mineral salts to a hot bath before bed.
✓ Eat foods high in vitamin E, including sunflower seeds, whole wheat, peanuts, cashews, almonds, walnuts, corn oil, soy oil, soy lecithin, spinach, asparagus, broccoli, oats, and avocados.
✓ Eat foods high in calcium, including cheddar, parmesan and romano cheeses, buttermilk, milk, yogurt, broccoli, kale, kelp, tofu, sardines, amaranth grain and flour, almonds, carob, brewer's yeast, sesame seeds, and teff.
✓ Eat foods high in vitamin C, including rose hips, acerola cherries, guavas, black currants, red peppers, oranges, grapefruit and other citrus fruits, cabbage, papayas, cantaloupe, and tomatoes.
✓ Eat foods high in vitamin D, including cod liver oil, eggs, herring, organ meats, salmon, and sardines.
✓ Eat foods high in magnesium, including blackstrap molasses, sunflower seeds, wheat germ, almonds, hazelnuts, Brazil nuts, pecans, walnuts, soybeans, soy lecithin, oats, barley, salmon, corn, avocados, bananas, cheese, tuna, and potatoes.
✓ Eat foods high in potassium, including bananas, cantaloupe, broccoli, avocados, Brussels sprouts, cauliflower, blackstrap molasses, brewer's yeast, brown rice, potatoes, legumes, dates, and whole grains.

And Try This!

Try relieving a cramp in the calf by standing with your feet flat on the floor and putting your full weight on the foot below the cramped calf. This is one of the ways professional athletic trainers treat them.

Did You Know?

The majority of the two hundred muscles that move the body, head, arms, legs, hands, feet, fingers, and toes work in opposing pairs. Certain muscles operate in concert. How efficiently we move through daily activity and perform our work depends on the orchestration of opposing and cooperating muscles.

Cystic Fibrosis

It is tempting to skip writing about a disorder that most medical authorities claim is incurable—cystic fibrosis (CF). However, some unconventional research suggests there is reason to revisit conventional opinion. Some years ago, Joel D. Wallach, a doctor of veterinary medicine working in the St. Louis Zoo under Dr. Marlin Perkins, performed an autopsy on a monkey that had died of an unknown cause. Dr. Wallach found the cause to be cystic fibrosis—and also something unexpected: the animal showed an acute deficiency in the trace mineral selenium.

Recognizing Cystic Fibrosis

Cystic fibrosis is most common among infants and children. Early symptoms may include the following:

- Sticky mucus in the lungs
- Frequent lung infections
- Heavy coughing and wheezing
- Breathing problems
- Digestive problems (especially with respect to fats)
- Malnutrition
- Excessive sweating
- Salty skin

What Are the Causes of Cystic Fibrosis?

Long considered an inherited disease, mainstream opinion has it that CF occurs when a defective gene from both parents causes cells that line the lungs to retain an abnormal amount of sodium and release too little chloride, making cells dry out and change normal lung mucus into a thick and sticky mass that's hard to cough up. Harmful bacteria thrive in this mucus and infect it, undermining the lungs, and cutting off oxygen and bringing early death for patients. A similar condition affects the pancreas, inviting a host of serious digestive disorders.

What You Can Take

Nutrients

Name	Dosage	Benefits
Vitamin A	10,000 IU daily	Deficiencies linked to cystic fibrosis.
Vitamin D	400 IU daily	Helps guard against lung infections.
Vitamin E	400 IU daily	Studies point to improvement among cystic fibrosis patients following supplementation.
Multivitamin and mineral complex	As directed on label	Helps prevent multiple deficiencies.
Manganese	5 mg daily	Enhances the effects of vitamin E.
Pancreatin	350–1,000 mg before each meal	Required for proper digestion of proteins.
Selenium	200 mcg daily	Deficiencies linked to cystic fibrosis. Studies point to improvement following supplementation.

What You Can Do

✓ Focus on nutritional supplements to cope with symptoms.
✓ Avoid mucus-causing foods such as dairy products.
✓ Avoid sugar and other refined carbohydrates.
✓ Avoid taking hydrochloric acid when ingesting pancreatic enzymes.

✓ Eat plenty of fresh fruits and vegetables.
✓ Eat foods high in vitamin A, including salmon, bass, halibut, mackerel, herring, whitefish, sardines, tuna, clams, shrimp, beef, chicken, pistachios, pecans, walnuts, lentils, and soybeans.
✓ Eat foods high in vitamin D, including cod liver oil, eggs, herring, organ meats, salmon, and sardines.
✓ Eat foods high in vitamin E, including sunflower seeds, whole wheat, peanuts, cashews, almonds, walnuts, corn oil, soy oil, soy lecithin, spinach, asparagus, broccoli, oats, and avocados.
✓ Eat foods high in selenium, including Brazil nuts, fish, organ meats, whole grains, eggs, cabbage, corn, peas, onions, garlic, chicken, beets, barley, and tomatoes.

And Try This!

Try eating mainly fresh fruits and vegetables, unprocessed nuts and seeds. Cooked and processed foods trigger the secretion of mucus. So do dairy products and meat.

Did You Know?

Another theory concerning the origin of cystic fibrosis is that it results from free radical attacks, an indirect way of saying that there are not enough antioxidants to control the free radicals. Some years ago, research at Johns Hopkins University School of Medicine demonstrated that a supplement of vitamin E improved symptoms associated with CF in children who had endured this condition for 10 years.

Cystitis
(Bladder and Urinary Tract Infections)

Almost every woman overcomes cystitis—bacterial infection of the bladder and/or urinary tract—and almost every woman gets it back, sometimes over and over again. Cystitis, although it can be highly uncomfortable, is not especially serious, but it can infect the kidneys and create major problems if left untreated. For this reason, antibiotics are often prescribed.

Recognizing Cystitis

Cystitis is far more common in women than men, but men do contract cystitis and can have a tough time getting rid of it. Symptoms may include:

- Frequent urination
- Feeling of having to urinate again right after you've gone
- Burning feeling during and following urination
- Cloudy urine with a strong odor
- Abdominal pain
- Blood in urine

Warning: See your doctor immediately if blood occurs in the urine.

What Are the Causes of Cystitis?

- Pregnancy
- Sexual relations
- Lack of fluids
- Bacteria from urethra (*E. coli* in 90 percent of cases)
- Vaginal secretions
- Waste matter contamination
- Abnormal blockages in the bladder or urethra
- Diet high in sugar and other refined carbohydrates
- Alcohol
- Diabetes

What You Can Take

Nutrients

Name	Dosage	Benefits
Vitamin A	25,000 IU daily for menopausal women and men; 10,000 IU daily for pregnant and pregnancy-eligible women	Stimulates the immune system to help fight off infection.
Vitamin C	500 mg three times daily	Stimulates the immune system to help fight off infection.
Probiotics (including acidophilus)	One capsule with up to 20 billion live cells twice daily	Helps recover from cystitis and build an army of friendly bacteria to defend against its return.
Zinc picolinate	15–30 mg daily	Speeds up healing, especially effective when taken with vitamin A.

Herbs

Name	Dosage	Benefits
Garlic (odorless)	Two capsules three times daily	Highly effective against bacterial infections.
Goldenseal	250 mg powdered extract three times daily	Kills *E. coli* and every other major microorganism that brings on cystitis.

What You Can Do

- ✓ Urinate frequently, especially before and after sex.
- ✓ Do not hold a full bladder.
- ✓ Drink at least 8–10 glasses of pure spring water daily.
- ✓ Drink 16 ounces of unsweetened cranberry juice daily or take 2 400 mg cranberry juice capsules daily.
- ✓ Avoid sugar and other refined carbohydrates.
- ✓ Avoid alcohol and caffeine.
- ✓ Exercise regularly.
- ✓ Work to relieve stress (*see* STRESS).

✓ Eat foods high in vitamin A, including eggs, milk, cheese, cream, butter, yogurt, salmon, bass, halibut, mackerel, herring, whitefish, sardines, tuna, clams, shrimp, beef, chicken, pistachios, pecans, walnuts, lentils, and soybeans.

✓ Eat foods high in vitamin C, including rose hips, acerola cherries, guavas, black currants, red peppers, oranges, grapefruit and other citrus fruits, cabbage, papayas, cantaloupe, and tomatoes.

✓ Eat foods high in zinc, including seafood, sardines, oysters, soybeans, soy lecithin, kelp, legumes, meat, liver, eggs, brewer's yeast, mushrooms, poultry, whole grains, and pumpkin and sunflower seeds.

✓ Use antibiotics sparingly unless infection spreads to kidneys.

And Try This!

Try taking a tablespoon of juniper berries in tea form added to a cup of boiling water, both when waking up and an hour before bed. It helps discharge more urine, acts as an antiseptic, and deodorizes the strong urine odor associated with cystitis with a floral scent.

Did You Know?

A study of 44 women and 16 men with cystitis by biochemist P. N. Podromos and associates demonstrated that 16 ounces of unsweetened cranberry juice daily brought marked benefits to 73 percent of those monitored.

Dandruff

Nobody has died from even the severest case of dandruff. So researchers across the globe are not going all out night and day to discover the best ways to prevent and manage it. However, a shoulder full of those unsightly white flakes is embarrassing. Fortunately, there are natural ways to banish dandruff.

Recognizing Dandruff

A common condition, the symptoms of dandruff are hard to miss:

- White flakes of dead skin on the scalp, shoulder, and/or clothes
- Itching and redness of the scalp (not always)

What Are the Causes of Dandruff?

- Nutritional deficiencies (especially biotin)
- Diet high in sugar and other refined carbohydrates
- Yeast overgrowth
- Poor digestion

What You Can Take

Nutrients

Name	Dosage	Benefits
Vitamin B-complex	100 mg daily	Biotin deficiency causes dandruff. Adequate supplementation combined with additional B vitamins can reverse condition.
Vitamin B_{12}	1,000 mcg under the tongue daily	Helps to reverse dandruff.
Vitamin E	400 IU daily	Helps to reverse dandruff.
Evening primrose oil	1,500 mg daily	Alleviates dry, itchy scalp.
Omega-3 essential fatty acids	1,000 mg softgel daily	Alleviates dry, itchy scalp.

What You Can Do

✓ Avoid sugar and other refined carbohydrates.
✓ Avoid fried foods.
✓ Avoid scratching itchy scalp, as it aggravates the condition.

✓ Eat plenty of fresh fruits and vegetables.
✓ Eat foods high in biotin, including brewer's yeast, meat, poultry, whole grains, soybeans, milk, and fish.
✓ Eat foods high in vitamin B_{12}, including liver, sardines, mackerel, herring, red snapper, flounder, salmon, lamb, Swiss cheese, blue cheese, eggs, haddock, beef, halibut, anchovies, chicken, turkey, milk, and butter.
✓ Eat foods high in vitamin E, including sunflower seeds, whole wheat, peanuts, cashews, almonds, walnuts, corn oil, soy oil, soy lecithin, spinach, asparagus, broccoli, oats, and avocados.
✓ Use Nizarol shampoo, an antifungal medication, if all else fails.

And Try This!

Try rinsing your hair with diluted lemon and vinegar after shampooing. It removes residue leftover from the shampoo and restores a healthy acid balance to the head.

Did You Know?

While affiliated with Queen Elizabeth College at the University of London, the noted nutrition researcher Dr. John Yudkin found that patients who ate the most refined sugar had the most dandruff, as reported in the *Encyclopedia of Common Diseases*. Double-checking his findings with more research, he then asked half of his patients with the worst cases of dandruff to continue eating their usual amounts of refined sugar, and the other half to stop eating it. A year later he found that, of the 11 patients permitted to continue eating their usual amount of sugar, 9 had the same extreme dandruff. Two were cured. Among the 8 non–sugar eaters, 7 were cured and the eighth showed improvement.

Depression

More than 10 million Americans suffer from some form of depression. And while psychologists and psychiatrists often engage in verbal warfare over which course of treatment is best, the one thing they can agree on is that there's a big difference between the blues and full-blown depression. The blues come and go, but depression hangs on. It dominates conduct and feelings for at least two consecutive weeks, and often for months or even years. Depressed individuals want to get out from under the weight of the world by trying anything reasonable that promises relief. Many turn to vitamins, minerals, and herbs—and results usually show they were wise to do so.

Recognizing Depression

- Sadness
- Despair
- Hopelessness
- Frequent tears
- Lack of interest in normal activities
- Sleep disorders (too much or not enough)
- Changes in appetite
- Muscle aches
- Fatigue
- Loss of self-esteem
- Inability to think clearly
- Thoughts of suicide

What Are the Causes of Depression?

- Nutritional deficiencies
- Chemical imbalances in the brain
- Physical illness
- Family history
- Low-protein diet
- Diet high in sugar and other refined carbohydrates
- Stress
- Low thyroid function
- Traumatic life events
- Lack of exercise
- Low blood sugar
- Food and environmental allergies

What You Can Take

Nutrients

Name	Dosage	Benefits
Vitamin B-complex	100 mg daily	Necessary for maintaining the biochemical balance of all B vitamins when supplementing with any single B vitamin individually.
Vitamin B_1	400 mg daily	Helps restore brain levels of the neurotransmitter acetycholine, a mood elevator.
Vitamin B_{12}	2,000 mcg daily	Needed for making BH4, the raw material for synthesizing antidepression neurotransmitters. Always supplement when taking high amounts of folic acid.
Vitamin C	1,000 mg three times daily	Needed for making BH4, the raw material for synthesizing antidepression neurotransmitters.
Folic acid	5 mg daily	Needed for making BH4, the raw material for synthesizing antidepression neurotransmitters.
L-tyrosine	1,500 mg after breakfast and lunch	Deficiencies linked to depression.
DL-phenylalynine	1,000 mg taken twice daily with L-tyrosine	Deficiencies linked to depression.
S-adenosyl methionine (SAMe)	400 mg twice daily for three weeks, then 200 mg daily for maintenance	Activates the brain to make the neurotransmitters serotonin and dopamine.

Herbs

Name	Dosage	Benefits
St. John's wort	300 mg (with 0.3 percent content of hypericum) three times daily	Decreases the speed at which the brain breaks down serotonin. Low levels of serotonin are associated with depression.

What You Can Do

✓ Test for low thyroid function (*see* HYPOTHYROIDISM).
✓ Test for food and environmental allergies (*see* ALLERGIES).
✓ Test for low blood sugar (*see* HYPOGLYCEMIA).
✓ Work to relieve stress (*see* STRESS).
✓ Avoid wheat, sugar, and other refined carbohydrates.
✓ Avoid alcohol and caffeine.
✓ Exercise daily.
✓ Eat foods high in tryptophan, including turkey, chicken, avocado, dairy products, bananas, dates, figs, kiwi fruit, mango, pecans, plums, tomatoes, and walnuts.
✓ Eat foods high in vitamin B_1, including brewer's yeast, broccoli, brown rice, Brussels sprouts, eggs, asparagus, fish, poultry, pork, whole grains, legumes, liver, peas, kelp, oatmeals, plums, prunes, raisins, and nuts.
✓ Eat foods high in vitamin B_{12}, including liver, sardines, mackerel, herring, red snapper, flounder, salmon, lamb, Swiss cheese, blue cheese, eggs, haddock, beef, halibut, anchovies, chicken, turkey, milk, and butter.
✓ Eat foods high in folic acid, including whole grains, wheat germ, bran, brown rice, liver, milk, beef, barley, chicken, tuna, salmon, lentils, legumes, brewer's yeast, cheese, oranges, mushrooms, and green leafy vegetables.
✓ Eat foods high in vitamin C, including rose hips, acerola cherries, guavas, black currants, red peppers, oranges, grapefruit and other citrus fruits, cabbage, papayas, cantaloupe, and tomatoes.
✓ Seek professional counseling if depression does not improve upon making nutritional and lifestyle changes.

And Try This!

Try spending more time outside on sunny days or in well-lit rooms. Studies suggest that bright light affects the pineal gland's production of melatonin, a hormone that is believed to help prevent depression.

Did You Know?

Disillusioned with conventional antidepressants, one-third to one-half of all patients with depression stop taking them due to mixed results and side effects such as blurred vision, drowsiness, insomnia, impotence, increased blood pressure, or weight gain.

Diabetes

Complications associated with diabetes are one of the nation's leading causes of death. The disease takes two forms: Type I and Type II. Roughly 10 percent of the diabetic population has Type I diabetes, also called juvenile diabetes. This name is inaccurate, as the inability to synthesize enough insulin for their needs is common in people up to age 30. Insulin-dependent diabetes is the more accurate name for this condition. Adult-onset diabetes (Type II) afflicts 90 percent of diabetics. Type II diabetics usually have enough insulin, but the body cells resist its action. Current estimates indicate that more than 6 million Americans suffer from diabetes.

Recognizing Diabetes

Although both types of diabetes differ, they are similar in that too much sugar is circulating in the blood. Symptoms are thus the same:

- Constant hunger and thirst (a demanding thirst is the most telltale sign of diabetes)
- Frequent need to urinate
- Weight loss
- Deep fatigue
- Depression
- Irritability
- Excessive itching (mainly among Type II diabetics)

What Are the Causes of Diabetes?

- Family history
- Diet too high in fats and too low in complex carbohydrates and fiber
- Nutritional deficiencies (especially chromium)
- Lack of exercise
- Overweight
- Stress
- Food allergies (especially dairy products and wheat)
- Viral infections (primarily Type I only)
- Low thyroid function

What You Can Take

Nutrients

Name	Dosage	Benefits
Vitamin B-complex	100 mg daily	Required for proper glucose metabolism.
Chromium	200 mcg daily	Lowers blood sugar levels by improving the efficiency of insulin.
Zinc	50 mg daily	Essential for normal insulin production.
Alpha lipoic acid	200 mg daily	Improves blood sugar control

Herbs

Name	Dosage	Benefits
Gymnema sylvestre	200 mg twice daily	Improves blood sugar control and can reduce the required amount of insulin.

What You Can Do

✓ Exercise daily (I suggest brisk walks for 30 minutes).
✓ Avoid sugar and other refined carbohydrates.
✓ Avoid alcohol (pure sugar!).
✓ Don't smoke.

✓ Avoid caffeine.
✓ Test for food and environmental allergies (*see* ALLERGIES).
✓ Maintain healthy body weight (*see* OVERWEIGHT).
✓ Work to relieve stress (*see* STRESS).
✓ Eat five or six small meals throughout the day as opposed to the standard three.
✓ Eat protein snacks between meals.
✓ Eat foods high in chromium, including brewer's yeast, broccoli, whole wheat, blackstrap molasses, mushrooms, nuts, barley, and thyme.
✓ Eat foods high in zinc, including seafood, sardines, oysters, soybeans, soy lecithin, kelp, legumes, meat, liver, eggs, brewer's yeast, mushrooms, poultry, whole grains, and pumpkin and sunflower seeds.

And Try This!

If you are a hypothyroid (get tested if you don't know and have diabetes), try taking a natural, desiccated thyroid supplement prescribed and tailored to your specific needs by a physician. Many diabetics suffer from undetected hypothyroidism, and studies have shown that desiccated thyroid can prevent, delay, and even reverse serious diabetic complications.

Did You Know?

A study by Dr. James Anderson, noted University of Kentucky biochemist, demonstrated that a fiber-rich, high-carbohydrate diet could help some diabetics free themselves from insulin shots. Dr. Anderson switched the diet of 13 diabetics, 8 on insulin and the other 5 on oral medications, from a high-fat diet with little fiber, to a regimen of 75 percent complex carbohydrates, 9 percent fat, and 20 grams of fiber. Within just 2 weeks, 4 of the 8 taking insulin were able to stop, and all 5 on oral medications were freed from them. Other insulin takers were able to reduce their dosages.

Diarrhea

Normally human wastes idle their way down the lower intestine, their fluids absorbed by the intestinal wall. They become formed by the bowel, and then casually exit from the body. Far from normal, diarrhea is an *emergency* situation! The body needs to get rid of something in a hurry and throws off unformed wastes and water. Diarrhea will usually run its course, yet there are things you can do to help it along.

Recognizing Diarrhea

- Bowels move too frequently
- Watery stools
- Stomach pain and cramping
- Excessive thirst
- Vomiting

What Are the Causes of Diarrhea?

- Contaminated food or water
- Intestinal bacteria or virus
- Yeast overgrowth
- Celiac disease
- Food and environmental allergies
- Stress

What You Can Take

Herbs

Name	Dosage	Benefits
Garlic (odorless)	1–3 tablespoons daily	Kills unfriendly bacteria that may cause diarrhea.

Homeopathy

Name	Dosage	Benefits
Colocynthis C	6c taken every three or four hours	Especially useful when diarrhea is accompanied by cramps.

What You Can Do

✓ Test for food and environmental allergies (*see* ALLERGIES).
✓ Avoid all dairy products.
✓ Avoid alcohol and caffeine.
✓ Avoid salads, local drinking water, and marginal restaurants when traveling in foreign countries. Drink bottled water.
✓ Increase intake of liquids to help flush out the system, including at least 8–10 glasses of pure spring water daily.
✓ Eat a pint of plain, cultured yogurt daily.
✓ Add fiber to the diet (oat bran is ideal).
✓ Take 2 tablespoons of carob powder daily.
✓ Work to relieve stress (*see* STRESS).

And Try This!

Try drinking a tea made of 2 tablespoons of blackberry bark or roots in 3 cups of water. Simmer it down to 2 cups and sip throughout the day.

Did You Know?

A study published in the *Canadian Medical Association Journal* reported that 253 children with diarrhea were fed a 5 percent solution of carob powder in rice water for 12–36 hours. Results showed that it required an average of 1.8 days to develop normal stools. This regimen was successful in 250 of the 253 cases. The researchers concluded, "Carob flour is unexcelled by any other pectin-based treatment that we have ever used."

Diverticulosis

Infrequent bowel movements cause waste matter to dry, harden, then break into hard pieces that put pressure on the tender intestinal membrane, making it bulge outward into small pockets where fecal matter collects, attracts harmful bacteria, and putrefies. This decay irritates and then inflames the sensitive membrane pockets, causing pain—a condition called diverticulitis. If left untreated, it may eventually require surgery.

Recognizing Diverticulosis

Diverticulosis is most prevalent among the elderly, but can affect those of all ages. Many people may be unaware they have the condition, as symptoms are not always prevalent, or may be confused with constipation. Other symptoms can include:

- Hard, dry stools that are difficult to pass
- Pain in lower abdomen
- Gas
- Cramps
- Bloating
- Indigestion

What Are the Causes of Diverticulosis?

- Constipation
- Diet low in fiber
- Stress
- Smoking
- Overweight
- Food allergies (especially dairy products and wheat)

What You Can Take

Nutrients

Name	Dosage	Benefits
Vitamin B-complex	100 mg daily	Helps heal gastrointestinal tract.
Vitamin C	500 mg three times daily	Softens the stool and encourages more frequent bowel movements. Helps heal the colon.
Multivitamin and mineral complex	As directed on label	Helps prevent pouches from forming.

| Acidophilus | Capsule with 1–2 billion live cells twice daily | Controls unfriendly bacteria in the lower intestine. |

Homeopathy		
Name	**Dosage**	**Benefits**
Nux vomica	Several 6c pellets twice daily	Promotes regularity.

What You Can Do

✓ Prevent or correct constipation before colon pockets are formed (*see* CONSTIPATION).

✓ Exercise regularly.

✓ Drink at least 8–10 glasses of pure spring water daily.

✓ Avoid sugar and other refined carbohydrates.

✓ Avoid processed foods.

✓ Eat plenty of whole foods that are high in fiber, including whole grains (if not wheat-intolerant), fresh fruits and vegetables, lentils, peas, and beans.

✓ Add fiber supplements such as chia seed (tablespoon dissolved in water) and psyllium (in water or juice) to the diet twice daily.

✓ Test for food allergies (*see* ALLERGIES).

And Try This!

Try taking 2 tablespoons of aloe vera juice three times daily. It increases regularity and helps heal the gastrointestinal tract.

Did You Know?

Diverticular disorders were almost unknown before 1900, when refined flour and sugar gained widespread use. Abram Hoffer, a pioneering nutrition-oriented medical doctor, notes that these disorders are rare in developing countries where fiber is an essential part of the daily diet. Dr. Hoffer estimates that, in the United States, 5 percent of everyone over 40 and two-thirds of the population over 80 develop diverticulosis.

Dizziness

Dizziness, sometimes called *vertigo* when the condition is extreme, is a loss of equilibrium that can occur due to many factors, but most often results from infections of the inner ear. Dizziness may also be a warning sign of more serious illness such as heart trouble or stroke, and should be brought to a doctor's attention when the underlying cause is not apparent.

Recognizing Dizziness

- Feeling light-headed
- Spinning sensation
- Faintness
- Inability to regain your balance

What Are the Causes of Dizziness?

- Infection of the inner ear
- Excessive earwax
- Decreased blood flow to the brain
- Fever
- Head injury
- Low or high blood pressure
- Low blood sugar
- Diabetes
- Anemia
- Heart arrhythmias
- Food and environmental allergies
- Nerve disorders
- Adrenal exhaustion
- Changes in air pressure (such as when flying)
- Reactions to antidepressants, antibiotics, diuretics, or tranquilizers

What You Can Take

Nutrients

Name	Dosage	Benefits
Beta-carotene	20,000 IU daily	Effective against inner ear infections, one of the primary causes of dizziness.
Vitamin C	500 mg three times daily	Effective against inner ear infections, one of the primary causes of dizziness.

Name	Dosage	Benefits
Selenium	100–200 mcg daily	Effective against inner ear infections, one of the primary causes of dizziness.

Herbs

Name	Dosage	Benefits
Garlic (odorless)	400 mg daily	Effective against inner ear infections, one of the primary causes of dizziness.
Ginger extract	100 mg every three hours, as required	Works quickly and decisively against dizziness.
Ginkgo biloba	80 mg three times daily	Increases blood flow to the brain.
Kelp	Tablet containing 225 mcg of iodine daily	Helpful in first-generation hypothyroids.

What You Can Do

✓ Avoid quick, jerky movements during bouts of dizziness.
✓ Avoid alcohol, caffeine, and salt.
✓ Don't smoke.
✓ Test for low thyroid function (*see* HYPOTHYROIDISM).
✓ Test for low blood sugar (*see* HYPOGLYCEMIA).
✓ Test for food and environmental allergies (*see* ALLERGIES).
✓ Check for excessive earwax or ear infection.
✓ Eat foods high in vitamin C, including rose hips, acerola cherries, guavas, black currants, red peppers, oranges, grapefruit and other citrus fruits, cabbage, papayas, cantaloupe, and tomatoes.
✓ Eat foods high in selenium, including Brazil nuts, fish, organ meats, whole grains, eggs, cabbage, corn, peas, onions, garlic, chicken, beets, barley, and tomatoes.

And Try This!
Try rising slowly from a nap or sleep. Blood pressure is reduced during such periods and can cause dizziness.

Did You Know?

Garlic is so highly regarded around the world for fighting infections (like those of the inner ear, which cause dizziness) that it is often referred to as "nature's antibiotic."

Dry Eyes (Sjögren's Syndrome)

Sjögren's syndrome, a condition more commonly known as dry eyes, is often associated with the autoimmune disease rheumatoid arthritis. The immune system can turn upon its own tissue and destroy the tear glands—opening the way for inflammation, infection, or ulcers of the cornea, the window of the eye.

Recognizing Dry Eyes

Dry eyes tend to appear more often in women then men, particularly after the onset of menopause. Symptoms include:

- Eyes that are constantly dry, gritty, and painful
- Inability to produce tears

What Are the Causes of Dry Eyes?

- Facial nerve damage
- Faulty arterial circulation of the eyes
- Nutrient deficiencies (especially vitamin A)
- Food and environmental allergies
- Contact lenses
- Exposure to cigarette smoke
- Marijuana use

What You Can Take

Nutrients

Name	Dosage	Benefits
Vitamin A	10,000–20,000 IU daily *Warning:* Pregnant or pregnancy-eligible women should take no more than 10,000 IU daily.	Required for proper functioning of all mucus membranes.
Vitamin B-complex	100 mg daily	Needed for food metabolism and feeding of the eyes.
Vitamin C	1,000 mg three times daily	Deficiencies linked to dry eyes.
Ginkgo biloba	60 mg three times daily	Increases blood circulation to the eyes, assisting in the production of tears.
Omega-3 fatty acids	1,000 mg capsule or softgel twice daily	Excellent lubricant for the eyes.

Herbs

Name	Dosage	Benefits
Bilberry extract	100 mg twice daily	Improves blood circulation to the eyes and strengthens capillaries.

What You Can Do

✓ Don't smoke tobacco or marijuana.
✓ Avoid exposure to secondhand smoke.
✓ Test for food and environmental allergies (*see* ALLERGIES).
✓ Eat foods high in vitamin A, including eggs, milk, cheese, cream, butter, yogurt, salmon, bass, halibut, mackerel, herring, whitefish, sardines, tuna, clams, shrimp, beef, chicken, pistachios, pecans, walnuts, lentils, and soybeans.
✓ Eat foods high in vitamin B$_6$, including brewer's yeast, brown rice, whole wheat, royal jelly, soybeans, rye, lentils, sunflower seeds, alfalfa, salmon, wheat germ, tuna, bran, wal-

nuts, cashews, peanuts, peas, liver, avocados, beans, turkey, oats, chicken, halibut, lamb, and bananas.

✓ Eat foods high in vitamin C, including rose hips, acerola cherries, guavas, black currants, red peppers, oranges, grapefruit and other citrus fruits, cabbage, papayas, cantaloupe, and tomatoes.

And Try This!

Try one of the treatments that's proved successful for my patients when supplementation alone failed to work: cutting out alcohol and caffeine, reducing sugar and salt intake, and drinking 8–9 glasses of water daily.

Did You Know?

In their book *Nutritional Medicine*, two English doctors, Stephen Davies and Alan Stewart, report on a Scottish study of 17 dry eye patients. After 2 months on nutritional supplements—3,000 milligrams of vitamin C and 50 milligrams of vitamin B_6 daily—10 of them showed marked improvement.

Ear Infections

Statistics scream as loudly as infants with painful ear infections that breastfeeding for at least the first 4 months of life minimizes or prevents earaches suffered by 92 percent of all children under 6. This makes many mothers whose babies have been bottle-fed wish they could put their lives on rewind, like a tape on the VCR.

Recognizing Ear Infections

Typical symptoms: infection, inflammation, and swelling of the inner ear, accompanied by fever, a runny nose, sore throat, earache, and irritability.

What Are The Causes of Ear Infections?

Ear fluid is blocked from flowing out of the Eustachian tube into the throat, due to:

* Allergy attack
* Upper respiratory infection
* Weak immunity in infants and young children
* Inflammation and swelling of the Eustachian tube opening

What You Can Take

Nutrients

Name	Dosage	Benefits
Vitamin A	5,000–10,000 IU daily for children; 25,000 IU daily for 2 weeks for adults, except pregnancy-eligible women, who are limited to 10,000 IU daily	Strengthens immunity.
Vitamin C	50 mg daily for children; 500 to 1,000 mg three times daily for adults	Strengthens immunity.
Flavonoids	50 mg daily for children; 100 mg three times daily for adults	Acts with vitamin C as an anti-inflammatory.
Zinc	5 mg daily for children for 10 days; 30 mg daily for adults for 30 days. Add 2 mg of copper daily after 30 days	Strengthens immune function and teams with vitamin A in fighting infections.

Herbs

Name	Dosage	Benefits
Echinacea	200 mg three times daily	Strengthens immune function.
Xylitol chewing gum	A stick three times daily	Reduces pressure in inner ear and may prevent infection.

What You Can Do

- ✓ Distract children in pain with a favorite activity.
- ✓ Have children in pain sit up to decrease blood flow to the head and reduce pressure on inflamed tissue.
- ✓ Use extra pillows under the child's head to relieve pain.
- ✓ Hold or secure a warm—not hot—heating pad to the ear.
- ✓ Yawn in the presence of the child in pain to induce him or her to yawn and reduce pressure on the inner ear.
- ✓ Ear drops—warm garlic, mullein-flower, lavender, or eucalyptus oil—should be used with guidance by a health professional.
- ✓ Refrain from using eardrops if the ear is draining.
- ✓ Eliminate suspect foods that may trigger allergy.
- ✓ Suspect low thyroid function if upper respiratory infections are frequent (*see* HYPOTHYROIDISM).
- ✓ Get a second opinion if relief from fluid pressure is suggested by means of a ventilation tube or by piercing the eardrum—both expensive and hazardous procedures.
- ✓ Refrain from inserting a cotton swab into the ear for fear of puncturing the eardrum.
- ✓ Beware of cleaning ears with hydrogen peroxide, an irritant to delicate ear tissue.
- ✓ Be sure to see a doctor if the ear pain comes with a fever above 101° F, a stiff neck, a splitting headache, and a leakage of fluid or pus from the ear.

And Try This!

Here's an old folk remedy for earache used in a number of African countries. You peel and roast a medium-size onion, cool it, place it in a clean cloth, and hold or secure it against your painful ear until the aching subsides.

Did You Know?

Alexander the Great not only subdued the Egyptians but also the earaches of his troops with a special Egyptian formula, writes Dian Dincin Buchman in *Ancient Healing Secrets*. You dice several peeled garlic cloves into half a cup of olive oil, leave it in a warm place for a few days, strain out the garlic, soak a small piece of clean cotton bandage in the concoction, and insert it into your sore ear, then wrap a warm scarf around your head to keep the ear warm.

Edema (Water Retention)

Edema is an excess buildup of fluids in the body, the fluids usually being a combination of water and salt. Also sometimes referred to as dropsy, one of my patients suffering from edema characterized the condition best: "I feel like a human sponge!"

Recognizing Edema

- Swelling and bloating (particularly in the legs and hands)
- Puffy eyes
- Weight gain
- Muscle aches
- Fatigue

What Are the Causes of Edema?

- Food and environmental allergies
- High blood pressure
- Stress
- Adrenal exhaustion
- Pregnancy
- Heart failure
- Cirrhosis of the liver
- Kidney malfunction
- Excessive salt or sugar intake
- Nutritional deficiencies
- Sodium and potassium imbalance

What You Can Take

Nutrients

Name	Dosage	Benefits
Vitamin A	25,000 IU daily *Warning:* Pregnant or pregnancy-eligible women should take no more than 10,000 IU daily.	Deficiencies can result in a buildup of excessive body fluid.
Vitamin B-complex	100 mg daily	Increases release of salt in the body.
Vitamin C	500 mg daily	Helps normalize exhausted adrenal glands.
Vitamin E	400 IU daily	Deficiencies can result in a buildup of excessive body fluid.
Pantothenic acid	200 mg daily	Increases release of salt in the body.
Taurine	500 mg three times daily on an empty stomach for a month	Helps restore the balance of sodium and potassium, and promotes the excretion of fluids.

What You Can Do

- ✓ Avoid alcohol and caffeine.
- ✓ Avoid sugar and other refined carbohydrates.
- ✓ Avoid salt, especially prevalent in processed foods.
- ✓ Avoid dairy products.
- ✓ Exercise regularly.
- ✓ Work to relieve stress (*see* STRESS).
- ✓ Test for food and environmental allergies (*see* ALLERGIES).
- ✓ Eat plenty of raw fruits and vegetables.
- ✓ Eat foods high in vitamin A, including eggs, milk, cheese, cream, butter, yogurt, salmon, bass, halibut, mackerel, herring, whitefish, sardines, tuna, clams, shrimp, beef, chicken, pistachios, pecans, walnuts, lentils, and soybeans.

✓ Eat foods high in vitamin C, including rose hips, acerola cherries, guavas, black currants, red peppers, oranges, grapefruit and other citrus fruits, cabbage, papayas, cantaloupe, and tomatoes.

✓ Eat foods high in vitamin E, including sunflower seeds, whole wheat, peanuts, cashews, almonds, walnuts, corn oil, soy oil, soy lecithin, spinach, asparagus, broccoli, butter oats, and avocados.

And Try This!

Try drinking a daily cup of tea made from dandelion root or leaves. It helps correct sodium and potassium imbalances associated with edema.

Did You Know?

Often prescribed by mainstream physicians, diuretics can relieve the pressure from edema, but they steal valuable minerals. They should only be used as a temporary measure until the basic causes of edema are found and eliminated.

Emphysema

Depending on whose statistics you accept, thirteen to fifteen times more smokers die of emphysema than nonsmokers. Get the picture? Emphysema is a chronic obstructive lung disease in which patients literally suffocate to death over time due to an inability to exhale properly. There is presently no known cure for emphysema, but there are things you can do to greatly relieve the condition and extend life. The first, of course, is to stop smoking—NOW!

Recognizing Emphysema

Some doctors rely on chest X-rays for an emphysema diagnosis. Unfortunately, X-rays do not show early signs of the disease, only advanced degeneration. A lung function test called the Forced Expiratory Volume is far more helpful, even in early cases. It measures the amount of air a person can forcefully exhale in one second. This varies according to height and weight. As an example, a six-foot-tall man who weighs 170 pounds should be able to exhale four liters of air in a second. Values below this serve as an early warning that emphysema is developing. Additional symptoms can include:

- Coughing (especially after strenuous physical activity)
- Shortness of breath
- Wheezing
- Mucus in the lungs

What Are the Causes of Emphysema?

Smokers and those whose parents, grandparents, or other close relatives were emphysema victims are most likely to develop this condition. Not only does smoking shrink arteries, limiting blood flow and the transporting of oxygen to the trillions of body and brain cells, but it introduces some 1,000 toxins into the lungs, among them carbon monoxide, which displaces the limited amount of oxygen available to emphysema victims.

What You Can Take

Nutrients

Name	Dosage	Benefits
Vitamin A	25,000 IU daily *Warning:* Pregnant or pregnancy-eligible women should take no more than 10,000 IU daily.	Helps keep mucus membranes in the lungs healthy and strengthens immune function.
Vitamin C	1,000 mg three times daily	Enhances the effects of vitamin E, important in keeping collagen healthy, and fights infection in the lungs.

Name	Dosage	Benefits
Vitamin E	800–1,200 IU daily	Antioxidant that protects cells from free radical damage, which is extremely important in cells of the lung air sacs.
Chlorophyll (liquid)	1 tablespoon twice daily	Soothes inflamed mucus membranes.
Germanium	200 mcg daily	Enhances tissue oxygenation and contributes to delaying deterioration of lung air sacs.
Lycopene	15 mg twice daily	Powerful antioxidant that protects the lungs from free radical damage.

What You Can Do

✓ Stop smoking at once. Seek professional help if you are unable to do so on your own.

✓ Avoid exposure to secondhand smoke and air pollution.

✓ Take the Forced Air Expiratory Volume test if you suspect that you are developing emphysema.

✓ Eat one or more serving of fresh fruit or vegetables with every meal.

✓ Avoid processed foods.

✓ Avoid mucus-forming foods such as dairy products and foods containing white flour.

✓ Eat foods high in vitamin A, including salmon, bass, halibut, mackerel, herring, whitefish, sardines, tuna, clams, shrimp, beef, chicken, pistachios, pecans, walnuts, lentils, and soybeans.

✓ Eat foods high in vitamin C, including rose hips, acerola cherries, guavas, black currants, red peppers, oranges, grapefruit and other citrus fruits, cabbage, papayas, cantaloupe, and tomatoes.

✓ Eat foods high in vitamin E, including sunflower seeds, whole wheat, peanuts, cashews, almonds, walnuts, corn oil, soy oil, soy lecithin, spinach, asparagus, broccoli, oats, and avocados.

And Try This!

Try sipping hot herbal tea to relieve the excessive mucus buildup that often accompanies emphysema.

Did You Know?

Estimates suggest that you lose 8 minutes off your life for every cigarette smoked. Do the math and you'll see that smoking is a deadly habit indeed!

Fatigue (Including Chronic Fatigue Syndrome)

A diagnosis that gives most doctors a headache that aspirin or feverfew can't relieve is fatigue, since it is generally a symptom of something else. Even more elusive is a form of severe and prolonged fatigue, which has come to be called chronic fatigue syndrome (CFS). CFS has been characterized as "tiredness multiplied by tiredness," and it is often accompanied by endless guilt about being nonproductive, depressed, and feeling worthless because family or companions are impatient with the patient's inability to recover, not realizing that the patient wants this more than anyone. Nothing turns a doctor into a detective quicker than trying to help such a person do so.

Recognizing Fatigue

Fatigue is a state of low energy or tiredness that interferes with a person's ability to function at a normal level. Everyone suffers from fatigue at times and to varying degrees, be it due to an underlying illness or simply burning the candle at both ends.

What distinguishes CFS from fatigue in general is the intensity and the duration of the fatigue (lasting for a minimum of 6 months), and the fact that no other underlying illnesses or other immediate cause can be identified as the source. CFS is often misdiagnosed if not ignored by members of the medical community, with many doctors still telling patients the problem is all in their heads. Anyone suffering from CFS knows this not to be the case. The condition is much more common in women than in men, especially in young adults under age 40. In addition to severe fatigue, symptoms associated with CFS can resemble the flu and may include the following:

- Sore muscle and joints
- Fever
- Sore throat
- Night sweats
- Swollen lymph nodes
- Profound depression

- Anxiety
- Headaches
- Irritability
- Mood swings
- Poor appetite
- Sleep problems

What Are the Causes of Fatigue?

Fatigue is a symptom of other disorders, not a medical condition as such. Contributing factors may include:

- Low thyroid function
- Low blood sugar
- Poor nutrition
- Lack of sleep
- Yeast overgrowth
- Anemia
- Food and environmental allergies
- Chronic infection

- Heart, kidney, or liver ailments
- Diabetes
- Overwork
- Stress
- PMS
- Adrenal exhaustion
- Drug use or reactions to prescription medications

Unlike fatigue in general, and despite some continued resistance, CFS is becoming more widely recognized as a medical condition in its own right. One major roadblock to CFS gaining larger acceptance has been the inability of experts to agree on what causes it. Some have linked it to viral infections, particularly the Epstein-Barr virus. Others believe it may have more to do with an inability to properly regulate blood pressure. Additional suspects include the following:

- Weakened immune and adrenal systems
- Nutritional deficiencies
- Multiple infections
- Mercury toxicity (mainly from dental fillings)

- Fibromyalgia
- Intestinal parasites
- Emotional factors
- Drug use or reactions to prescription medications

What You Can Take

Nutrients

Name	Dosage	Benefits
Vitamin B-complex	100 mg daily	Necessary for maintaining the biochemical balance of all B vitamins when supplementing with any single B vitamin.
Vitamin B$_{12}$	1,000 mcg under the tongue daily	Widely used treatment for low energy.
Vitamin C	1,000 mg three times daily	Deficiencies linked to CFS.
Vitamin E	400–800 IU daily	Deficiencies linked to CFS.
Carnitine	500 mg daily	Drives fat through cell membranes and into the mitochondria. Promotes weight loss and enhances enzymes essential to metabolizing carbohydrates.
Coenzyme Q-10	50 mg twice daily	Ignites metabolism to produce energy in all cells and fights free radicals.
Magnesium	400 mg daily	Essential to creating energy. Deficiencies produce symptoms of muscle weakness and fatigue.
Medium-chain triglycerides	Five 100 mg capsules or two or more spoonfuls daily	Absorbed by the liver for an instantly recallable energy reserve.
Nicotinamide adenine	2.5 mg daily or up to 5 mg a week later, if	Highly active molecule that delivers energy to the cells and

Name	Dosage	Benefits
dinucleotide hydride (NADH)	response is not satisfactory	increases stamina.
Octacosanol	40–80 mg daily	Natural energy booster derived from wheat germ oil.
Taurine	2 g daily	Increases stamina.
Trimethylglycine	5 mg daily	Fatigue fighter used by athletes to increase endurance.
Shark liver oil	500 mg capsule twice daily	Used for centuries by Scandinavians to increase energy levels and for a host of other health concerns.
Adrenal extract	500 mg crude factor daily	Helps restore adrenal exhaustion.
Thymus extract	750 mg crude factor daily	Boosts immunity.
Desiccated liver	Three 10 grain tablets after each meal	Increases energy levels.

Herbs

Name	Dosage	Benefits
Panax ginseng	100–250 mg daily	Increases energy, boosts immunity, stabilizes blood sugar, and fights free radicals.
Siberian ginseng (dried root)	2–4 g daily	Used by athletes to increase energy and is especially effective for patients with CFS.

What You Can Do

✓ Exercise daily.
✓ Get plenty of rest.
✓ Avoid sugar and other refined carbohydrates.
✓ Avoid drugs, alcohol, and caffeine.
✓ Test for low thyroid function (*see* HYPOTHYROIDISM).
✓ Test for food and environmental allergies (*see* ALLERGIES).
✓ Test for low blood sugar (*see* HYPOGLYCEMIA).

✓ Work to relieve stress (*see* STRESS).

✓ Drink at least 8–10 glasses of pure spring water daily.

✓ Eat 1 teaspoonful of wheat germ oil daily.

✓ Eat plenty of raw fresh fruits and vegetables.

✓ Eat foods high in vitamin B_{12}, including liver, sardines, mackerel, herring, red snapper, flounder, salmon, lamb, Swiss cheese, blue cheese, eggs, haddock, beef, halibut, anchovies, chicken, turkey, milk, and butter.

✓ Eat foods high in vitamin C, including rose hips, acerola cherries, guavas, black currants, red peppers, oranges, grapefruit and other citrus fruits, cabbage, papayas, cantaloupe, and tomatoes.

✓ Eat foods high in vitamin E, including sunflower seeds, whole wheat, peanuts, cashews, almonds, walnuts, corn oil, soy oil, soy lecithin, spinach, asparagus, broccoli, butter oats, and avocados.

✓ Eat foods high in magnesium, including blackstrap molasses, sunflower seeds, wheat germ, almonds, hazelnuts, Brazil nuts, pecans, walnuts, soybeans, soy lecithin, oats, barley, salmon, corn, avocados, bananas, cheese, tuna, and potatoes.

And Try This!

Try soaking a tablespoon of chia seeds in a glass of water and drink daily. You can also add it to oatmeal or whole grain hot cake mix. The Aztecs in southernmost North America grew and used chia seeds to sustain good health and supercharge their energy and endurance. Native Americans of what is now the Southwest region of the United States harvested chia seeds from plants that grew wild. It was one of their major foods.

Did You Know?

Even some modern-day alternative doctors forget about a standard nutritional supplement that, for decades, supercharged human energy and stamina. This is desiccated liver made from raw animal liver that's defatted, defibered, and then dried. Because it is not heated in these processes, it remains loaded with vitamins and minerals. Its unique power to energize us and extend our endurance was dramatically demonstrated in an experiment conducted some years ago by Dr. B. H. Ershoff. One of two groups of mice on the same diet received desiccated liver for several weeks. When both groups were placed in separate swimming tanks, the mice that weren't fed the desiccated liver supplement could swim only 13 minutes to total exhaustion. Three mice on desiccated liver swam 63, 83, and 87 minutes—about five to eight times longer! Nine other mice fed this supplement astonished the researchers by continuing to swim vigorously after 2 hours when the test was concluded.

Fibromyalgia

One of my fibromyalgia patients, a 27-year-old assistant purchasing agent for an electronics firm, let it all hang out about her symptoms: "My fatigue is so sapping that I have to flog myself to go to work. At night, I just fall into bed with my clothes on. I sleep poorly, because my muscles and bones feel as if someone had driven an ice pick into them. When the bedsheet touches tender points on my back, my butt, elbows, knees, neck, rib cage, and thighs, I want to scream." She wasn't exaggerating!

Recognizing Fibromyalgia

Fibromyalgia is a condition of generalized muscle pain (severe at times) with no immediately detectable cause. All areas of the body may suffer, but pain is most often felt in the head, back, legs, and chest, and frequently takes the form of what are called tender points. It is much more common in women than in men. Additional symptoms may include:

- PMS
- Dizziness
- Depression

- Sleep disorders
- Fatigue
- Anxiety
- Irritable bowel and/or bladder
- Poor coordination

What Are the Causes of Fibromyalgia?

There is no generally agreed-upon cause of fibromyalgia, but experts point to the following factors as likely contributors:

- Low thyroid function
- Low blood sugar
- Stress
- Depression
- Lack of exercise
- Food and environmental allergies
- Weak immune system
- Yeast overgrowth
- Anemia

What You Can Take

Nutrients

Name	Dosage	Benefits
Vitamin C	1,000 mg three times daily	Protects muscle cells against free radical damage.
Grape seed extract	100 mg three times daily	Protects muscle cells against free radical damage.
Magnesium	300–600 mg daily (taken together with malic acid)	Reduces pain, increases energy levels, and serves as a muscle relaxant.
Malic acid	1,200–2,400 mg daily (taken together with magnesium)	Reduces pain, increases energy levels, and serves as a muscle relaxant.
Melatonin	3 mg an hour before bedtime	Helps promote sleep.

Name	Dosage	Benefits
S-adenosyl-methionine (SAMe)	200 mg intramus-cularly and 400 mg orally twice daily	Reduces pain.
Thyroid hormone	As prescribed by a physician	Low thyroid function has been linked to fibromyalgia.

Herbs

Name	Dosage	Benefits
St. John's wort	300 mg three times daily	Effective against depression and increases pain toler-ance.

What You Can Do

✓ Test for low thyroid function (*see* HYPOTHYROIDISM).
✓ Test for low blood sugar (*see* HYPOGLYCEMIA).
✓ Test for food and environmental allergies (*see* ALLERGIES).
✓ Reduce stress (*see* STRESS).
✓ Don't smoke.
✓ Avoid alcohol and caffeine.
✓ Avoid sugar and other refined carbohydrates.
✓ Drink at least 8–10 glasses of pure spring water daily.
✓ Exercise regularly.
✓ Get enough rest.
✓ Eat plenty of fresh fruits and vegetables.
✓ Eat foods high in vitamin C, including rose hips, acerola cherries, guavas, black currants, red peppers, oranges, grapefruit and other citrus fruits, cabbage, papayas, cantaloupe, and tomatoes.
✓ Eat foods high in magnesium, including blackstrap molasses, sunflower seeds, wheat germ, almonds, hazelnuts, Brazil nuts, pecans, walnuts, soy beans, soy lecithin, oats, barley, salmon, corn, avocados, bananas, cheese, tuna, and potatoes.

And Try This!

Try taking cold showers in the morning. Studies suggest they can help alleviate muscle pain associated with fibromyalgia.

Did You Know?

Dr. Guy Abraham conducted a double-blind study of 15 patients from 32 to 60 years of age. Within 48 hours of receiving a dose ranging from 1,200 to 2,400 mg of malic acid—found in apples—and 300 to 600 mg of magnesium daily, all 15 patients reported far less pain in tender points. Eight weeks later the pain was almost gone.

Food Poisoning

It's not fair! Armies of invisible, poisonous, food-borne bacteria can undermine you before you're even aware of them. However, with some uncommonly good common sense, you can level the playing field—no, the battlefield!

Recognizing Food Poisoning

The signs of food poisoning are:

- Abdominal cramps
- Dehydration
- Diarrhea
- Intestinal gas
- Nausea
- Vomiting

What Are the Causes of Food Poisoning?

- Contaminated foods or water
- Unclean hands of food preparers
- Unsanitary food preparation conditions—cutting boards, sinks, kitchen towels used too long without thorough washing, germ-laden sponges and abrasive cloths
- Cracked dishes or cups where germs congregate
- Refrigerators and freezers set at too high temperatures
- Foods insufficiently cooked
- Raw fish, rare steaks
- Deficient home canning practices

What You Can Take

Nutrients

Name	Dosage	Benefits
Vitamin A	10,000 IU daily	Helps heal irritated stomach and intestinal linings.
Vitamin C	500 mg three times daily	Helps heal damaged gastro-intestinal membranes.
Zinc	30 mg daily	Contributes to healing.
Probiotics (including acidophilus)	Up to 20 billion organisms daily	Manages diarrhea, implants friendly bacteria in the colon.
Charcoal powder	1/4 cup thoroughly stirred in a glass of water every three hours	Helps control vomiting and diarrhea and absorbs gas.
Burned toast (if no charcoal is available)	One slice every three hours	Helps control vomiting and diarrhea and absorbs gas.

Herbs

Name	Dosage	Benefits
Carob powder	5 percent solution in water, twice daily	Combats vomiting and diarrhea.
Ginger	200 mg capsule daily	Helps overcome nausea.
Goldenseal	500 mg twice daily	Fights bacterial infection—including *E. coli*.

What You Can Do

✓ Be wary of picnic potato salad, Caesar salad made with raw eggs, and chiffon pie!

✓ Don't eat, cook, or bake with eggs with cracked shells.

✓ Refrain from eating fish, meat, or poultry stored in the refrigerator for 4 or more days.

✓ Make sure your refrigerator cools at or below 40° F and your freezer goes no higher than O° F.

✓ Refrigerate hot foods immediately, rather than letting them cool at room temperature.

✓ Don't let juices from refrigerated raw meat, fish, or poultry drip on foods beneath them.

✓ Thaw frozen foods in the refrigerator, rather than at room temperature. (This includes turkeys.)

✓ Wash countertops or cutting boards with warm water and soap—especially after cutting up raw poultry—before further use.

✓ Always use a plastic cutting board, rather than a wooden one that's more subject to indentations where harmful bacteria lodge.

✓ Scrub vegetables before eating!

✓ If food poisoned, don't force vomiting by putting fingers down your throat. Nature will control your vomiting.

✓ Drink additional water when food-poisoned to avoid dehydration.

✓ Resume the intake of food with easy-to-digest clear soups and herbal tea.

✓ Eat two to three slices of plain bread to soak up poisons.

✓ Drink only spring water or filtered tap water.

✓ When eating out, always choose a sparkling, clean restaurant that exhibits an "A" certificate near the rest room. ("B" is a passing grade in school, but not in restaurants.)

✓ See a doctor if diarrhea, cramping, and vomiting don't stop within 24 hours.

✓ See a doctor if blood appears in your vomit or stool.

And Try This!
Three homeopathic remedies help food poisoning:

1. Arsenicum album at 6c or 12c strength every 3 hours, if you vomit, have diarrhea and feel cold and restless.
2. Veratrum album at 6c or 12c potency every 3 hours, if you experience cold sweats and want cold beverages in addition to showing the major symptoms.
3. Carbo vegetabilis at 6c or 12c strength every 3 hours if you are weak, sweaty, bloated, and flatulent along with the major symptoms.

Did You Know?

Ancient Romans, Arabs, and Egyptians ate the sweet and yellow carob pulp—especially when they suffered digestive disturbances such as diarrhea. To cope with infant diarrhea, carob powder, diluted in water or milk, has been used in the United States since the early 1950s.

Foot Problems

All the short and long muscles of the foot and leg helped primitive people adjust to varying terrain. Some historians of physiology maintain that in today's cities feet can't work normally. Unyielding sidewalks, streets, wood or tile floors, and tight rigid shoes have essentially changed the feet from gripping appendages to slabs of flesh and bones like hooves. Obviously, we don't want to abolish sidewalks, paved streets, and tile floors. However, our ability to adapt to hard surfaces has not been ideal—and our feet often pay the price.

Recognizing Foot Problems

Like shoes, foot problems come in all shapes and sizes. The most common include the following:

Bunions

Bunions are a swelling of the inner side of the big toe. This forces the big toe to the outer side of the foot, creating greater friction, swelling, and inflammation over the big toe and its bursa, the insulation sac between bone and skin. Bunions typically result from jogging and wearing narrow shoes (especially high heels). Surgical removal, a relatively minor procedure, is the standard treatment.

Corns

Corns are small painful overgrowths of horny skin with a central core. They are caused by tight-fitting shoes. Collodion, an over-the-counter solution, applied to corns for several nights softens them. Then soaking them in hot water makes them removable.

Neuromas

Neuromas are tumors on nerve ends between the toes, especially prevalent in joggers, runners and others who spend hours on their feet. The five metatarsal bones in the forefoot and toe bones pinch the nerves between the toes. Symptoms include burning, numbness or sharp pins and needles that sometimes even radiate upward to the leg. Neuromas should be treated by a podiatrist or medical doctor.

Heel Spurs

Heel spurs occur when the ligament on the bottom of the foot pulls away from the heel. This leads to deposits of sharp calcium on the bone that rasp the flesh with each step. Heel spurs don't disappear magically. A podiatrist has to perform surgery on them.

Toenail Fungus

Toenail fungus is best thought of as athlete's foot gone underground. Even with strong drugs such as Lamisil and Sporonox, it can be extremely hard to get rid of, taking a minimum of three to nine months. The best natural approach is tea tree oil. Undiluted tea tree oil should be rubbed on the nail and area around it twice daily, followed by application of the penetrant DMSO (available in health food stores) that carries the oil through the nail to the fungus. I also suggest taking two aged garlic capsules (300 mg) twice daily. Be patient, results may take just as long as with conventional drugs, but you'll be spared the side effects.

Athlete's Foot

Athlete's foot is an annoying fungal infection on the feet and between the toes, causing itching, redness, cracked skin, swelling, and scaling. The fungus thrives in damp and warm places like communal showers. Recommended treatments are provided later in this section.

What Are the Causes of Foot Problems?

In addition to the information already noted concerning specific conditions, poor-fitting shoes, hard surfaces, and exercise are what keep podiatrists (foot doctors) in business.

What You Can Take (Athlete's Foot Only)

Nutrients

Name	Dosage	Benefits
Vitamin A	10,000 IU daily	Speeds up healing of athlete's foot.
Vitamin C	500 mg three times daily	Speeds up healing of athlete's foot.
Zinc	30 mg daily	Speeds up healing of athlete's foot.

Herbs

Name	Dosage	Benefits
Aged garlic (Kyolic)	Two capsules twice daily after breakfast and dinner	Highly effective against athlete's foot.

What You Can Do

In General

✓ Run, if you must, on soft-surface high school or college running tracks, rather than on hard sidewalks or streets. I recommend walking instead.

✓ Use the right kind of shoes for all athletic activities (e.g. don't jog in shoes designed for basketball). Avoid low-cost shoes made from synthetic materials that can cause athlete's foot and rashes.

✓ Get help from a podiatrist for bunions, corns, neuromas, heel spurs, toenail fungus, and other foot injuries.

For Athlete's Foot Prevention

✓ Keep your feet, socks, and the inside of your toes dry.

✓ Go barefoot and wear open sandals so perspiration can readily evaporate.

✓ Air out shoes after wearing them.

✓ Wear sandals in indoor swimming pools, in athletic club showers, or on carpeting of hotel and motel rooms.

For Athlete's Foot Infection

✓ Apply tea tree oil two to three times daily to affected areas.

✓ Add 20–25 drops of tea tree oil to a basin of warm water and soak your feet for 15–20 minutes to shorten the healing period.

✓ Apply garlic oil or dust affected areas with garlic powder (if garlic is too powerful, it can be diluted with almond oil).

✓ Apply aloe vera to affected areas.

✓ Spread calendula lotion or cream thinly on affected areas.
✓ Soak feet in solution of half apple cider vinegar and half water.

And Try This!

Try soaking tired feet in several quarts of warm water spiked with two or three tea bags. The tannin in tea helps fight bacteria and fungi that can cause athlete's foot and other rashes. It also relieves fatigue and relaxes the feet.

Did You Know?

In addition to the foot problems noted here, long-distance runners on hard pavement often suffer serious injury, not unlike cross-country truck drivers who take such a pounding that they sometimes sustain kidney ailments. Some years ago I read an article in the *New England Journal of Medicine* reporting on how habitual joggers experience so much jarring of the bladder that they occasionally show blood in their urine.

Frostbite

It usually surprises patients headed for cold country to go skiing or ice fishing when I suggest they take liberal amounts of vitamin C to protect themselves. Most know that vitamin C can work minor miracles with many ailments, but frostbite? One patient, an ad agency executive, phoned me after a remote area ski resort experience to say: "Thanks for the vitamin C tip, Doctor. I did what you suggested, and I was comfortable while most of the guys with me complained about the cold."

Recognizing Frostbite

- Hard, white skin on the areas of the body affected, those most vulnerable generally include the hands, feet, face, and ears
- Affected areas of skin may begin to peel within a day or two
- Loss of feeling in affected areas
- Swelling, itching, and pain may occur once affected area is warmed up
- Affected areas of skin may remain highly sensitive to cold long after condition has been treated

Warning: If frozen extremities turn black, get qualified help immediately. This is a medical emergency.

What Are the Causes of Frostbite?

Frostbite occurs when any area of the body is exposed to extreme cold. A foot falling through the ice of a frozen pond would be a good example.

What You Can Take

Nutrients

Name	Dosage	Benefits
Vitamin C	500 mg three times daily when traveling in cold country	Offers protection against frostbite when taken prior to cold weather exposure.

What You Can Do

- ✓ Treat frostbitten hands or feet with circulating warm water or warm air—not snow or ice water.
- ✓ Apply aloe vera to frozen fingers or toes to relieve pain and promote healing.
- ✓ Eat foods high in vitamin C prior to cold weather exposure, including rose hips, acerola cherries, guavas, black currants, red peppers, oranges, grapefruit and other citrus fruits, cabbage, papayas, cantaloupe, and tomatoes.

And Try This!

Try the homeopathic remedy agaricus. Two pellets of 30c taken every half hour usually bring positive results in the form of preventing tissue damage and accelerated healing.

Did You Know?

Investigating the medicinal benefits of aloe vera, Dr. John P. Heggers and associates at the University of Texas Medical Branch at Galveston treated frostbite with aloe vera and conventional salves, ointments, and oils. The team found that frostbite-injured skin treated with aloe vera healed with much less tissue damage than that treated with the usual remedies.

Gallstones

Like many other organs, the 4-inch-long, pear-shaped gallbladder, positioned between your liver lobes, is not a thing of beauty. Nor is it a joy forever—particularly when it develops gallstones that can double you over with pain.

However, it does a necessary job: storing and concentrating liver-manufactured bile (another name for gall) and releasing bile into the small intestine so that you can digest fat or fat-soluble vitamins such as A, D, E, or K. Gallstones can be the size of a pinhead or as large as a golf ball.

Recognizing Gallstones

A pain in the upper right abdomen that grows increasingly sharp is an early warning of gallstones. As the gallbladder becomes inflamed and swells, you develop a fever and a queasy stomach and may throw up. Don't treat such an attack lightly. It can be deadly.

What Are the Causes of Gallstones?

A green fluid, bile, composed of calcium, phospholipids, fatty acids, and water, is the material from which gallstones are formed. Trouble starts in the gallbladder when there is too little lecithin or bile acid in relation to cholesterol. Elevated cholesterol in the gallbladder—there's no relation to blood cholesterol levels—crystallizes, attracts more cholesterol, and causes the formation of a gallstone that plugs the bile duct. Other causes:

- A low-fiber diet
- A high intake of saturated fat
- Drinking less than 7–8 glasses of water a day
- Food allergies

What You Can Take

Nutrients

Name	Dosage	Benefits
Vitamin C	1,000 mg three times daily	Lowers cholesterol, particularly in the bile.
Taurine	1,000 mg two times daily	Enhances ability to dissolve existing stone and improves bile flow.
Lecithin	1,200 mg capsule twice daily	Homogenizes fat, helping to prevent crystallizing of bile.
Fiber (psyllium seed or oat bran)	5–10 g daily	Helps prevent constipation, a possible contributor to gallstones.

Herbs

Name	Dosage	Benefits
Milk thistle (Silybum marianum)	200 mg (70% content of silymarin) twice daily	Keeps bile liquid to minimize stone formation.
Peppermint oil (enteric-coated capsule)	One to two 0.2 ml capsules three times daily	Helps dissolve gallstones.

What You Can Do

✓ Drink at least 8 glasses of water daily.
✓ Add more vegetables to the diet for fiber.
✓ See ALLERGIES for detection methods to minimize chance of allergies.
✓ Beware of fasting or extreme calorie restriction, which can contribute to gallstone formation.
✓ Minimize or eliminate coffee, which may cause gallbladder to contract.
✓ Avoid smoking. It narrows arteries and may cause gallbladder contraction.
✓ Avoid a high intake of refined sugar, a risk factor for gallstones.
✓ Remember that gallstones can be removed by conventional allopathic medicine means: surgery, dissolved by allopathic medicines, or shattered ultrasonically.

And Try This!

Try the Breneman diet for gallstones that eliminates these foods: apricots, beef, beet, cherry, peach, rice, rye, soy, and spinach. All 69 patients who refrained from these foods for from 3 to 5 days were free of gallstone symptoms. Symptoms returned when they reintroduced these foods into their diets.

Did You Know?

A study of 206 fair-skinned people who enjoyed sunbathing revealed them to be at twice the risk of developing gallstones as those who disliked sunbathing. Alarming is the fact that those who always burn after long sunbathing are at twenty times the risk of developing gallstones as those who don't care for sunbathing.

Gas (Intestinal)

One of those subjects that no one's supposed to talk about—intestinal gas—should be discussed in order to find physiological solutions that will make the world a better place. Inasmuch as intestinal gas is a topic of more than passing interest, let's deal with the stressors, allergens, and foods that cause it and the best ways to banish it.

Recognizing Gas

Recognizing gas is usually not a problem, either for you or (unfortunately) sometimes those around you. Common symptoms include:

- Foul-smelling wind
- Abdominal cramping
- Bloating
- Belching
- Bad breath
- Rumbling sounds in the stomach

What Are the Causes of Gas?

Stressors of all kinds make eaters scarf their food too fast and secrete too little stomach acids, bile, and digestive enzymes for the proper breakdown of proteins into amino acids, complex carbohydrates into simple sugars, and fats into fatty acids and glycerol. Other factors that can cause gas include the following:

- Constipation
- Food allergies and intolerances (especially to dairy products and wheat)
- Foods such as beans, lentils, grains, Brussels sprouts, cabbage, cauliflower, corn, dried fruit, eggs, pistachio nuts, pumpkin, and fried foods
- Diets too high in fiber
- Carbonated beverages
- Not chewing food properly
- Drinking too many liquids with meals (weakens digestive enzymes)

What You Can Take

Nutrients

Name	Dosage	Benefits
Charcoal (activated)	500 mg after each meal or every two hours, if needed	Absorbs gas and deodorizes it.
Hydrochloric acid	648 mg of betaine hydrochloride and 130 mg of pepsin	Helps normalize digestion, minimizing gas.

Herbs

Name	Dosage	Benefits
Garlic (odorless)	1 teaspoon after meals	Increases the production of gastric juices, stimulating the movement of wastes out of the lower intestine so putrefactive bacteria have little chance to create gas; and reduces the size of gas bubbles.
Fennel	Half a teaspoon after each meal	Increases the production of gastric juices, stimulating the movement of wastes out of the lower intestine so putrefactive bacteria have little chance to create gas; and reduces the size of gas bubbles.

What You Can Do

✓ Relieve stress (*see* STRESS).

✓ Eat slowly and make sure to chew food completely.

✓ Limit the amount of liquids consumed with meals.

✓ Test for food allergies (*see* ALLERGIES).

✓ Prepare beans so that they become less offensive by soaking them in a pot, bringing them to boil, emptying the water, and then adding new water for cooking.

✓ Test for sufficient hydrochloric acid in the stomach if you digest food poorly.

✓ Limit intake of milk at any one time to reduce gas. Substitute with lactase-containing milk or yogurt.

✓ Take Beano, a tasteless brown liquid that often relieves gas caused by beans and lentils, among other foods.
✓ Avoid alcohol, caffeine, and carbonated beverages.
✓ Avoid antacids to relieve gas, as they often make matters worse.

And Try This!

Try starting each meal with a slice of pineapple. Pineapple contains the enzymes bromelain and papain, both of which are important for proper digestion and can help prevent gas.

Did You Know?

Lactobacillus acidophilus in yogurt makes its own lactase, so most milk intolerants can enjoy yogurt, which also serves another purpose: implanting friendly bacteria in the colon that helps digestion.

Gingivitis

During World War I, troops on the front lines developed gum tenderness, inflammation, and swelling (occasional bleeding), a condition so prevalent that it was called Trench Mouth, or Vincent's disease to those in the dental profession. Prevailing opinion held that it was caused mainly by wartime conditions—not enough time or inclination to brush teeth regularly, poor personal hygienic practices, and passing highly infectious germs from one soldier to another due to crowded facilities. Probably all of these conditions contributed to gingivitis (inflamed gums). Yet there was still another. In the years since then, it was found that stress diminishes immune system defense against harmful organisms, many of which are directly related to the condition.

Recognizing Gingivitis

- Red, swollen, and inflamed gums
- Bleeding gums
- Painful gums (sometimes)

What Are the Causes of Gingivitis?

- Plaque that sticks to the teeth
- Poor dental hygiene
- Poor dental work (e.g. loose fillings, dental implants that don't fit correctly)
- Brushing teeth too hard
- Stress
- Nutritional deficiencies (especially vitamin C)
- Diet high in sugar and other refined carbohydrates
- Smoking

What You Can Take

Nutrients

Name	Dosage	Benefits
Vitamin A	50,000 IU daily for a week, but only with approval and monitoring by your doctor or dentist *Warning:* Pregnant or pregnancy-eligible women should take no more than 10,000 IU daily.	Helpful in both preventing and correcting gingivitis, especially when taken together with vitamin E.
Vitamin C (with bioflavonoids)	500 mg of vitamin C and 250 mg of bioflavonoids three times daily	Deficiencies can result in scurvy and related gum disease. Supplementation has also been found helpful in healing gingivitis.
Vitamin E	400 IU daily	Helpful in both preventing and correcting gingivitis, especially when taken together with vitamin A.
Coenzyme Q-10	50 to 70 mg daily	Has shown phenomenal healing powers in gum ailments.

Zinc picolinate	15–30 mg daily	Essential to proper healing of gingivitis, especially when taken together with vitamin A.

Herbs

Name	Dosage	Benefits
Echinacea and goldenseal	300 mg of echinacea and 50 mg of goldenseal daily	Highly effective in reversing gingivitis.

What You Can Do

✓ Avoid over-the-counter products that promise to cope with gingivitis.
✓ Practice good oral hygiene (brush with warm water and make sure to floss daily).
✓ See your dentist every 6 months.
✓ Don't smoke.
✓ Avoid alcohol.
✓ Avoid sugar and other refined carbohydrates.
✓ Apply aloe vera to inflamed gums.
✓ Drink 8–10 glasses of pure spring water daily.
✓ Relieve stress (*see* STRESS).
✓ Eat foods high in vitamin A, including eggs, milk, cheese, cream, butter, yogurt, salmon, bass, halibut, mackerel, herring, whitefish, sardines, tuna, clams, shrimp, beef, chicken, pistachios, pecans, walnuts, lentils, and soybeans.
✓ Eat foods high in vitamin C, including rose hips, acerola cherries, guavas, black currants, red peppers, oranges, grapefruit and other citrus fruits, cabbage, papayas, cantaloupe, and tomatoes.
✓ Eat foods high in vitamin E, including sunflower seeds, whole wheat, peanuts, cashews, almonds, walnuts, corn oil, soy oil, soy lecithin, spinach, asparagus, broccoli, oats, and avocados.
✓ Eat foods high in coenzyme Q-10, including salmon, sardines, mackerel, and spinach.
✓ Eat foods high in zinc, including seafood, sardines, oysters, soybeans, soy lecithin, kelp, legumes, meats, liver, eggs, brewer's yeast, mushrooms, poultry, whole grains, and pumpkin and sunflower seeds.

And Try This!

Try applying goldenseal powder to gums with your fingers. I've seen patients conquer gingivitis in little more than 2 weeks when combining this treatment with daily supplements of goldenseal and echinacea in pill form.

Did You Know?

Edward Wilkinson, a dentist in the U.S. Air Force, did some of the significant early research on coenzyme Q-10, approaching the study with admitted prejudice. He called himself a "top-notch skeptic on Co Q-10." Giving gingivitis patients 50 to 70 mg daily, he soon saw amazing reversals of the condition, changes he "could hardly believe."

Glaucoma

Glaucoma is characterized by a gradual and painless buildup of fluid in the eye. Pressure on the optic nerve brings on tunnel vision and then blindness. Conventional medicine offers drugs that reduce the pressure. However, this delaying action does not correct the basic problem.

Recognizing Glaucoma

Open-angle glaucoma (90 percent of all cases) is most prevalent in those over 40 and rarely exhibits symptoms until the condition is very well advanced. Warning signs at this point may include:

- Poor or complete loss of peripheral vision
- Poor night vision
- Too frequent need to change eyeglass prescription
- Headaches

What Are the Causes of Glaucoma?

- Nutritional deficiencies
- Stress
- Food and environmental allergies
- Family history
- Diabetes
- High blood pressure
- Eye injuries

What You Can Take

Nutrients

Name	Dosage	Benefits
Vitamin C	2,000 mg daily	Important to the integrity of collagen. Blockage of the eye comes from a deterioration of collagen.
Magnesium	250 mg daily	Relaxes eye muscles, enriches blood supply, and increases the visual field.

What You Can Do

- ✓ Have an eye test at least twice a year (especially if you detect any loss in peripheral vision).
- ✓ Test for food and environmental allergies (*see* ALLERGIES).
- ✓ Work to relieve stress (*see* STRESS).
- ✓ Eat fish twice a week or take a tablespoon of cod liver oil every other day.
- ✓ Don't smoke.
- ✓ Avoid alcohol and caffeine.
- ✓ Eat foods high in vitamin C, including rose hips, acerola cherries, guavas, black currants, red peppers, oranges, grapefruit and other citrus fruits, cabbage, papayas, cantaloupe, and tomatoes.
- ✓ Eat foods high in magnesium, including blackstrap molasses, sunflower seeds, wheat germ, almonds, hazelnuts, Brazil nuts, pecans, walnuts, soybeans, soy lecithin, oats, barley, salmon, corn, avocados, bananas, cheese, tuna, and potatoes.

And Try This!

Try taking regular breaks (every half hour if possible) when engaged in activities that are stressful to the eye such as staring at a computer screen for extended periods of time. Reducing such stress can help prevent glaucoma.

Did You Know?

Biochemist Prasad S. Kulkarni, of the University of Louisville, got an idea that cod liver oil might work from an observation that Eskimos have low rates of glaucoma. He wondered if this might be due to the fact that their diet is rich in fish and fish oils. Dr. Kulkarni followed his hunch by testing it on rabbits, soaking their food in cod liver oil. These were normal rabbits without glaucoma; however, their intraocular pressure dropped by an average of 56 percent. Once off this diet, the rabbits' eye pressure returned to normal.

Gout

I had treated the husband of the patient across the desk from me for gout, one of the most excruciating kinds of arthritis, and casually mentioned that 95 percent of sufferers from this ailment are men. "Ninety-five percent," she replied. "That's too bad. The other five percent deserves it, too!"

Recognizing Gout

Actually, nobody deserves gout. If it afflicts women at all, it is usually after menopause. Gout usually attacks the joint of your big toe at night when you're sound asleep. However, it may strike other joints as well, including the knees, wrists, and hands. It comes with chills and fever. Gnawing pain is so sharp that even lightweight bedding adds to the torture.

What Are the Causes of Gout?

There's little mystery as to what causes gout and how it brings pain. Usually overweight people who underexercise and overeat certain types of food—purine-rich anchovies, sardines, herring, mackerel, organ meats such as liver, and shellfish—either produce a buildup of uric acid in the bloodstream or can't throw off enough and deposits form in the joints. Contributing factors include:

- Alcohol
- Stress
- Injury
- Nutritional deficiencies

What You Can Take

Nutrients

Name	Dosage	Benefits
Vitamin E	400–800 IU daily	Reduces inflammation and fights free radicals.
Eicosapentaenoic acid (EPA)	300 mg twice daily or in an omega-3 formula containing 200 mg of docosahexaenoic acid (DHA)	Reduces the amount of uric acid in the blood, and decreases inflammation as well as the possibility of tissue damage.
Folic acid	800–1,600 mcg daily *Warning:* This is a large dose. Inasmuch as more than usual amounts of folic acid can mask symptoms of vitamin B-$_{12}$ deficiency, it is advisable to take 1000 mcg of B$_{12}$ daily as well.	Limits the enzyme that activates the production of uric acid.
Quercetin	250 mg three times daily	Blocks pain-promoting inflammatory substances associated with gout.

Herbs

Name	Dosage	Benefits
Bromelain	250–500 mg three times daily between meals and 250 mg daily when symptoms start to recede	An enzyme derived from pineapple that increases recovery time from gout.

What You Can Do

✓ Maintain ideal body weight (*see* OVERWEIGHT).

✓ Relieve stress (*see* STRESS).

✓ Avoid foods with a high purine content such as anchovies, sardines, herring, mackerel, shellfish, and organ meats such as liver.

✓ Avoid alcohol.

✓ Avoid high-fat foods.

✓ Avoid sugar and other refined carbohydrates.

✓ Drink at least 8–10 glasses of pure spring water daily.

✓ Exercise regularly.

✓ Increase consumption of complex carbohydrates, including plenty of fresh fruits and vegetables, whole cereals, brown rice, bulgar wheat, barley and bran, chickpeas, and beans and lentils.

✓ Eat foods high in vitamin E, including sunflower seeds, whole wheat, peanuts, cashews, almonds, walnuts, corn oil, soy oil, soy lecithin, spinach, asparagus, broccoli, oats, and avocados.

✓ Eat foods high in folic acid, including whole grains, wheat germ, bran, brown rice, milk, beef, barley, chicken, tuna, salmon, lentils, legumes, brewer's yeast, cheese, oranges, mushrooms, and green leafy vegetables.

And Try This!

Try eating cherries. And not only because they taste good—they work! I suggest no less than half a pound per day combined with a daily pint of cherry juice. If you're not able to eat that many cherries every day, try cherry fruit extract pills (1,000 mg daily) available in health food stores.

Did You Know?

Gout is commonly referred to as "the rich man's disease" because it is primarily the result of a diet high in fatty foods, meats, and alcohol.

Headaches and Migraines

Headaches come in all shapes and sizes, from a mild one brought about by skipping your second cup of morning coffee to an excruciatingly painful migraine induced by an allergic reaction or low blood sugar. And regardless of the severity, impatient patients want to know how to rid themselves of the pain—*now!*

Recognizing Headaches and Migraines

In the vast majority of headaches (*tension headaches*), arteries in the head constrict then swell abnormally and press on sensitive nerves, resulting in the constant, muscle-tightening pain around the head we normally associate with headaches.

Cluster headaches, however, are different. They get their name from the fact that there is often a clustering of as many as twenty headache attacks daily for months. Pain concentrates only on one side of the head, and can last for minutes or hours.

Migraines are far more than just a bad headache and much less common, accounting for less than 10 percent of all headaches. They make the head throb mercilessly with pain—usually on just one side—and the gut ache. Accompanying symptoms are often similar to those of seasickness and include:

- Dizziness
- Vomiting
- Diarrhea
- Cold hands
- Blurred vision

What Are the Causes of Headaches and Migraines?

- Food and environmental allergies
- Stress
- Anxiety
- Depression
- Caffeine withdrawal
- Fluctuating estrogen levels
- Low blood sugar
- Lack of magnesium
- Eye strain
- Dehydration (cause of hangover headaches)
- Vertebral misalignment
- Sinus infections
- Dental problems
- Constipation
- Overexertion
- Smoking

What You Can Take

Nutrients

Name	Dosage	Benefits
Vitamin B-complex	100 mg daily	Necessary for maintaining the biochemical balance of all B vitamins when supplementing with any single B vitamin individually.
Vitamin B$_2$	400 mg daily	Reduces the number of migraines endured by chronic sufferers.
Magnesium	300–400 mg daily	A fast-acting and highly effective mineral treatment for headache and migraine relief.
5-HTP	100 mg twice daily	Converts to serotonin, a brain neurotransmitter that produces pain-relieving effects.

Herbs

Name	Dosage	Benefits
Feverfew	250 mg three times daily	Reduces migraine pain, nausea, and vomiting.
Ginger (powdered)	Mix a half teaspoon in hot water, cool, strain, then drink when headache starts.	Effective headache reliever.

What You Can Do

✓ Test for food and environmental allergies (*see* ALLERGIES).
✓ Allergists and clinical ecologists report that the foods most responsible for triggering headaches and migraines include beef, cheeses, chocolate, corn, milk, eggs, oranges, pork, rye, wheat, soy, shellfish, yeast, potatoes, and coffee.
✓ Even more troublesome are foods high in additives, particularly nitrites, nitrates, benzoic acid, sulfur dioxide, and yellow and red dyes. Foods to watch out for in this category include bacon, ham, hot dogs, salami, and most dried fruits.
✓ Tyramine is the most notorious dietary ingredient causing migraines. It does so by dilating brain blood vessels that impinge on sensitive nerves. Common foods and beverages containing tyramine include beer, red wine, bananas, cheeses, chicken livers, citrus fruit, coffee, pickled fish, raisins, and sausages.
✓ Eat breakfast to prevent low blood sugar (*see* HYPOGLYCEMIA).
✓ Exercise regularly.
✓ Alternate warm and cold showers or foot baths.
✓ Relieve stress (*see* STRESS).
✓ Wean yourself off caffeine gradually.
✓ Consume fluids before bed following a night of drinking to prevent dehydration (better yet, don't drink!). Also try eating fruits and vegetables in advance.
✓ Always read under proper light.
✓ Avoid constipation (*see* CONSTIPATION).
✓ Avoid reliance on aspirin and other over-the-counter painkillers, as they can make frequent headaches worse over time.
✓ Eat foods high in magnesium, including blackstrap molasses, sunflower seeds, wheat germ, almonds, hazelnuts, Brazil nuts, pecans, walnuts, soybeans, soy lecithin, oats, barley, salmon, corn, avocados, bananas, cheese, tuna, and potatoes.

And Try This!

Try listening to music. A one-year study of migraine patients conducted at California State University at Fresno found that listening to soft, soothing music reduced the number of migraines experienced sixfold.

Did You Know?

Researchers in the University of Wisconsin biodynamics lab found that by walking or running for 30 minutes 3 days weekly, migraine sufferers reduced their attacks by 50 percent.

Hearing Loss

This is an age of noise pollution that includes many ear-shattering contributions: the clatter of jackhammers, the deafening smash of metal-forming machines in industrial plants, blasts of dynamite to remove rock, explosions of fireworks, earth-shaking artillery fire, screaming sirens, and the roar of jet planes during takeoffs and landings. As many as 30 million Americans suffer from some form of hearing loss, and exposure to loud noise is enemy number one. Earplugs can protect us from expected and repetitive noises. However, many come at us unexpectedly.

Recognizing Hearing Loss

Hearing loss can develop gradually over an extended period of time like that commonly associated with getting older, or suddenly such as that brought about by an infection or excess earwax. Sudden losses are usually quite obvious and are often accompanied by pain. However, in cases of gradual loss the symptoms can easily go undetected, and are frequently noticed first by others. Warning signs may include the following:

- Speaking too loudly (like that of someone talking with headphones on)
- Leaning toward a sound with one ear (favoring one ear over another)
- Regularly asking for things to be repeated
- Keeping volume levels on the TV or stereo too high without realizing it

What Are the Causes of Hearing Loss?

- Super-loud music and noises
- Nutritional deficiencies
- Impaired blood circulation
- Aging
- Inherited structural problems
- Severe ear accidents
- Excessive ear wax
- Bacterial and viral infections
- Food and environmental allergies (especially dairy products and wheat)
- Smoking
- Diabetes
- High blood pressure

What You Can Take

Nutrients

Name	Dosage	Benefits
Vitamin A	20,000 IU daily for 2–3 weeks, then 10,000 IU daily for several months *Warning:* Pregnant or pregnancy-eligible women should take no more than 10,000 IU daily.	Deficiencies cause an overgrowth and hardening of small inner ear bones, and have been linked to deafness.
Vitamin B-complex	100 mg daily	Necessary for maintaining the biochemical balance of all B vitamins when supplementing with any single B vitamin individually.
Vitamin B_{12}	1,000 mcg under the tongue daily	Provides protection against hearing loss due to loud noise exposure.

Name	Dosage	Benefits
Vitamin D	400 IU daily	Helps maintain the proper concentration of calcium in the inner ear fluid, and strengthens the main bones in the inner ear.
Ginkgo biloba	40 mg daily	Promotes blood circulation in the ears, essential to proper hearing.
Iodine	225 mcg daily taken in the form of a kelp pill	Deficiency linked to hearing loss.
Magnesium	400 mg daily	Provides protection against hearing loss due to loud noise exposure.
Niacin	100 mg daily in addition to the B-complex vitamins	Promotes blood circulation in the ears, essential to proper hearing.

What You Can Do

- ✓ Minimize exposure to loud music and noise.
- ✓ Wear earplugs when such exposure is unavoidable.
- ✓ Keep ears free of earwax by cleaning regularly.
- ✓ Test for food and environmental allergies (*see* ALLERGIES).
- ✓ Don't smoke.
- ✓ Avoid caffeine and alcohol.
- ✓ Eat foods high in vitamin A, including eggs, milk, cheese, cream, butter, yogurt, salmon, bass, halibut, mackerel, herring, whitefish, sardines, tuna, clams, shrimp, beef, chicken, pistachios, pecans, walnuts, lentils, and soybeans.
- ✓ Eat foods high in vitamin D, including cod liver oil, eggs, herring, organ meats, salmon, and sardines.
- ✓ Eat foods high in magnesium, including blackstrap molasses, sunflower seeds, wheat germ, almonds, hazelnuts, Brazil nuts, pecans, walnuts, soybeans, soy lecithin, oats, barley, salmon, corn, avocados, bananas, cheese, tuna, and potatoes.

And Try This!

Try adhering to the following rule of thumb: Any time you need to raise your voice to be heard over background noise such as the TV or stereo, your surroundings are too loud and could be contributing to future hearing loss. Such conditions are not always avoidable, but you'll be surprised how often they may be of your own making.

Did You Know?

To protect the hearing of 300 recruits on 2 months of basic training in a simulated combat area with battlefield artillery firing, military doctors gave half the group 167 mg of magnesium aspartate in a drink each day and the other half a look-alike placebo. Recruits taking magnesium showed less potential for permanent hearing loss than those on the placebo. The researchers consider magnesium useful protection when it's not practical to use earplugs.

Heart Attack

Heart attacks kill more than half a million Americans every year. A troubling statistic to be sure, but the dramatic nature of a heart attack itself can be even more frightening. We've all heard stories about someone suddenly dropping dead one day without warning. Medically defined as a myocardial infarction, a heart attack occurs when the blood supply to the heart is cut off or severely restricted, depriving it of oxygen.

Recognizing a Heart Attack

A large percentage of heart attacks strike with little or no indication they were coming. Symptoms that suggest you could be suffering from a heart attack include the following:

* Severe chest pain that may spread to the left side of the body, mainly the left arm, face, and neck
* Pain may last for several hours prior to a heart attack or occur suddenly
* Irregular heartbeats (arrhythmias)
* Sweating
* Trouble breathing
* Dizziness
* Nausea

Warning: Get to a hospital immediately upon experiencing the first signs of a heart attack. This is a medical emergency where seconds count.

What Are the Causes of Heart Attack?

A heart attack generally occurs for one of several reasons. The first is that an irregular heartbeat or series of them that may weaken the pumping action of the heart to a degree that it is unable to provide itself with enough blood. Another is that internal bleeding can prevent enough blood from flowing to the heart. The most frequent cause of a heart attack results from an artery becoming blocked, usually due to a blood clot and to the fact that the arteries have become narrow from a slow buildup of plaque (arteriosclerosis). Factors known to contribute to the risk of heart attack include:

* Low thyroid function
* Stress
* Overexertion
* Overweight
* Family history
* Smoking
* Drug or alcohol abuse
* High blood pressure
* High cholesterol
* Diabetes
* Lack of exercise
* Nutritional deficiencies (especially magnesium)

What You Can Take

Nutrients

Name	Dosage	Benefits
Vitamin E	400 IU daily	Improves circulation and reduces the risk of blood clots.
Coenzyme Q-10	100 mg daily for 12 weeks	Increases the strength of heart pumping action.
L-carnitine	1,000–2,000 mg daily	Increases the strength of heart pumping action.
Magnesium	400–1,000 mg daily	Prevents irregular heartbeats.

Herbs

Name	Dosage	Benefits
Liquid garlic (odorless)	1 teaspoon three times daily	A natural blood thinner.

What You Can Do

✓ Exercise regularly, but don't overdo it.
✓ Relieve stress (*see* STRESS).
✓ Test for low thyroid function (*see* HYPOTHYROIDISM).
✓ Drink at least 8–10 glasses of pure spring water daily.
✓ Don't smoke.
✓ Avoid drugs, alcohol, and caffeine.
✓ Avoid sugar and other refined carbohydrates.
✓ Maintain a health body weight (*see* OVERWEIGHT).
✓ Eat a handful of walnuts daily.
✓ Eat foods high in vitamin E, including sunflower seeds, whole wheat, peanuts, cashews, almonds, walnuts, corn oil, soy oil, soy lecithin, spinach, asparagus, broccoli, and avocados.
✓ Eat foods high in magnesium, including blackstrap molasses, sunflower seeds, wheat germ, almonds, hazelnuts, Brazil nuts, pecans, walnuts, soybeans, soy lecithin, oats, barley, salmon, corn, avocados, bananas, cheese, tuna, and potatoes.
✓ Eat foods high in coenzyme Q-10, including salmon, sardines, mackerel, and spinach.

And Try This!

Try drinking several cups of green tea daily. It is low in caffeine, loaded with antioxidants, and dozens of studies point to its effectiveness in preventing heart disease, cancer, and other serious ailments.

Did You Know?

Several years ago, a comprehensive study of 22,071 male physicians revealed that men five feet seven inches tall or shorter are 60 to 70 percent more likely to experience a heart attack than men over six feet one inch tall. Similar patterns have been found in women.

Heartburn and Hiatal Hernia

Hiatal hernia is a common condition where the upper part of the stomach bulges upward through the diaphragm into the esophagus, often caused by straining during bowel movements. Heartburn accompanies hiatal hernia, and is characterized by stomach acid then flowing upward into the esophagus, also referred to as acid reflux. Nearly 50 percent of the U.S. population experiences heartburn and hiatal hernia at some point during their lives.

Recognizing Heartburn and Hiatal Hernia

- Burning pain in chest and/or stomach
- Gas
- Belching
- Difficulty swallowing

What Are the Causes of Heartburn and Hiatal Hernia?

- Strained bowel movements and constipation
- Low-fiber diet
- Lack of exercise
- Coffee
- Alcohol
- Carbonated beverages
- Spicy foods
- Fried foods
- Ulcers
- Stress

What You Can Take

Nutrients

Name	Dosage	Benefits
Vitamin B-complex	100 mg twice daily	Improves digestion.

Herbs

Name	Dosage	Benefits
Aloe vera juice	Half-cup three times daily between meals	Soothes inflamed esophagus.
Gamma-oryzanol	100 mg three times daily between meals	Improves function of digestive tract.
Ginger	25–40 drops of tincture in one-third cup water	Relaxes walls of esophagus.
Licorice deglycyrrhizinated (DGL)	400 mg three times daily	Helps repair the stomach's mucus lining.

What You Can Do

- ✓ Exercise daily.
- ✓ Avoid constipation (*see* CONSTIPATION).
- ✓ If symptoms are common at night, do not eat within several hours of going to bed.
- ✓ Eat fiber-rich foods such as asparagus, raspberries, strawberries, cucumbers, cauliflower, whole grain cereals and bread, and brown rice.

✓ Eat slowly and chew food completely.
✓ Drink at least 8–10 glasses of pure spring water daily.
✓ Don't smoke.
✓ Avoid alcohol and coffee.
✓ Avoid spicy foods, fried foods, and foods high in fat.
✓ Avoid carbonated beverages.
✓ Relieve stress (*see* STRESS).
✓ Try sleeping in a more reclined position, rather than flat.

And Try This!

Try sipping the following formula that was created by Dr. Robert Downs, director of the Southwest Center of the Healing Arts in Albuquerque, New Mexico: 1 part aloe vera juice mixed with 4 parts of papaya juice and a matching part of sugar-free ginger ale or club soda. Dr. Downs and his hiatal hernia patients swear by it!

Did You Know?

A simple way to relieve heartburn is to chew a stick of sugarless gum. This gives rapid relief. Why? Chewing the gum enhances the production of saliva that carries stomach acid away.

Hemorrhoids (Piles)

Most people call them hemorrhoids. Others call them by their older name: piles. But both groups call them everything from annoying to itching to downright painful. There's no full agreement as to what hemorrhoids are. General opinion holds that they are enlarged varicose veins—internal or external—in the rectum, the last five inches of the large intestine ending at the anus, the exit for waste matter.

Recognizing Hemorrhoids

More than half of all Americans have experienced hemorrhoids to some degree. Common symptoms include:

- Swelling and inflammation of the rectum
- Rectal pain
- Rectal itching
- Rectal bleeding

What Are the Causes of Hemorrhoids?

Most medical literature states that, in addition to the strain of evacuating impacted fecal matter during constipation, heavy lifting, overweight, and the ordeal of labor in delivering a baby can overstress, enlarge, and sometimes rupture these engorged hemorrhoids. Other contributing factors include:

- Low-fiber diet
- Lack of exercise
- Lack of fluids
- Overuse of laxatives
- Sitting for long periods of time
- Food allergies

What You Can Take

Nutrients

Name	Dosage	Benefits
Vitamin A	10,000 IU daily	Good tissue healer, especially when taken together with zinc.
Vitamin C	500 mg three times daily	Softens stools, encourages bowel movements, and helps correct capillary fragility.
Flavonoid compound	Four to six 100 mg capsules daily	Reduces bleeding and pain associated with hemorrhoids.
Psyllium (powdered soluble fiber)	1 tablespoon with fruit or juice daily	Softens stools and encourages bowel movements.
Zinc	15–30 mg daily (if taken for longer	Good overall healer, especially when taken together

Name	Dosage	Benefits
	than thirty days, add 2 mg of copper each day)	with vitamin A.

Herbs

Name	Dosage	Benefits
Butcher's broom	150 mg capsule three times daily	Strengthens capillaries and arteries, and may help shrink enlarged veins.

What You Can Do

✓ Avoid constipation (*see* CONSTIPATION).
✓ Avoid sitting for long periods without a break.
✓ Drink at least 8–10 glasses of pure spring water daily.
✓ Eat a fresh fruit or vegetable with each meal.
✓ Exercise for 30 minutes daily after dinner.
✓ Use the softest possible bathroom tissue on bleeding hemorrhoids.
✓ Avoid heavy lifting.
✓ Avoid laxatives.
✓ Test for food allergies (*see* ALLERGIES).
✓ Maintain ideal body weight (*see* OVERWEIGHT).

And Try This!

Try taking a cool 15-minute sitz bath in the morning and before bedtime. When the rectal area is clean, gently apply 1 of 4 salves or ointments: St. John's wort, calendula, goldenseal, or aloe vera. Three to 4 applications daily help. St. John's wort seems most effective for itching. However, all of them encourage rapid healing.

Did You Know?

Remarkable success with internal and external hemorrhoids has been scored by Dr. Bernard A. L. Wissmer of the University of Geneva in Switzerland. After a week on a daily regimen of 4 to 6 100 mg capsules of bioflavonoid compound—rutin derived from buckwheat and hesperidin from citrus peels—250 patients started to heal. Then he lowered the intake to 2 to 3 capsules for three to four more weeks, and their bleeding and pain stopped. Dr. Wissmer reports that thousands of his patients have been relieved of hemorrhoids with his protocol.

Hepatitis

The liver's near miraculous ability to regenerate itself is severely tested by both the mild and severe forms of liver inflammation, from virus-caused hepatitis A and hepatitis B. Although hepatitis A usually destroys liver cells for a month or more, hepatitis B can destroy them for many months—or without stopping. Both kinds impair the liver's ability to handle carbohydrates, to synthesize bile to digest fat, and to remove toxins and waste.

Recognizing Hepatitis

It's not easy to recognize hepatitis from symptoms, because many of its symptoms are typical of other ailments—particularly flu-like symptoms: abdominal distress, drowsiness, fever, headache, jaundice (sometimes), loss of appetite, muscle soreness, nausea, and vomiting. Otherwise more obvious symptoms include liver tenderness and dark urine, plus abnormal lab results: low white blood cell count, a sharply elevated level of the liver enzyme aminotransaminase, and high levels of bilirubin, a reddish-yellow ingredient in blood and bile.

What Are the Causes of Hepatitis?

For hepatitis A:

- Contaminated food, water, or other beverages
- Unsanitary cooking and food handling
- Unclean public bathrooms

For hepatitis B:

- Virus transmitted through saliva or through semen or vaginal secretions during sexual contact
- Infected hypodermic needles
- Blood transfusions

What You Can Take

Nutrients

Name	Dosage	Benefits
Vitamin C	1,000 mg three times daily	Slowly relieves symptoms of viral hepatitis.
Vitamin C (megadoses)	40–100 g daily for acute viral cases, monitored by a doctor	Manages symptoms of viral hepatitis more rapidly.
Vitamin E	400 IU daily	Teams with vitamin C as antioxidant protection for the liver.
Liver extracts	100 mg three times daily	Helps liver to regenerate.
Alpha-lipoic acid	200 mg three times daily	Serves as an antioxidant in water *and* fat and enhances potency and life of vitamins C and E.

Herbs

Name	Dosage	Benefits
Licorice	200 mg (22% glycirrhyzinic acid) three times daily for two weeks	Protects liver by its antioxidants and antiviral action.
Milk thistle (silymarin)	100 mg four times daily for six–twelve months	Helps reverse liver damage and normalize its function.
Dandelion root	500 mg two to three times daily	Blocks liver damage and promotes its healing.

What You Can Do

✓ Practice extreme caution and hygiene in dealing with hepatitis patients. All forms are contagious until 3 weeks to a month after their onset.
✓ Spend almost full time in bed if you have hepatitis.
✓ Suspend work in places of contact with people until the contagious period has passed.
✓ Replace lost body fluids with vegetable juices (diluted by half with spring water).
✓ Sip vegetable broth and herbal teas throughout the day.
✓ Eat only natural foods.
✓ Totally avoid simple carbohydrates (refined sugar and flour), saturated fats, and fried foods.
✓ Stick to a high-fiber diet!
✓ After feeling better, slowly resume normal activities.
✓ Avoid strenuous exercise.
✓ Don't smoke.
✓ Don't drink alcohol.
✓ Prevent use of harsh chemicals in and around the home to ease the burden on your liver.

And Try This!

Try a cup of green tea three times daily. This is an old Russian remedy for infectious diseases, including hepatitis.

Did You Know?

Green, yellow, and orange cantaloupes are an excellent fresh fruit with which to start breakfast. However, they're more than that in China. Eaten several times a day, they are considered a pleasant means of coping with the symptoms of hepatitis.

Hiccups

One of those trivial but annoying ailments is hiccups, described in the *American Heritage Dictionary* as "a spasm of the diaphragm resulting in a sudden, abortive inhalation that is stopped by a spasmodic glottal closure." Well, maybe a professor of physiology will understand this—especially if he or she has experienced hiccups.

Recognizing Hiccups

It is hard not to recognize hiccups, a persistent noise made by diaphragm spasms that cause a closing of the glottis, the elongated space between the vocal cords.

What Are the Causes of Hiccups?

Even experts in physiology are not certain what causes them. However, they believe that they are brought on by eating or drinking too fast.

What You Can Take

The negligible amount of research conducted for hiccups offers no clue as to any nutrient that can prevent or alleviate this condition. However, a great number of folk medicine procedures that may be helpful are listed below.

What You Can Do

There's little scientific agreement as to how you get hiccups, so let's move on to something more important: how to get rid of them. Here are a dozen ways, most of them solidly based on the science of folk medicine. Supposedly, they shut off nerve impulses or increase the blood level of carbon dioxide.

✓ Soak a lemon slice in angostura bitters, then suck on it (you may not like the taste, but neither will your hiccups).

✓ Place in your mouth a level tablespoon of peanut butter—preferably from organically grown peanuts—and swallow it slowly. By the time it's gone, your hiccups should be gone, too.

✓ Chew a teaspoonful of mint leaves.

✓ Make a tea of catnip and sip it slowly. Your cat may join you—even if he or she has no hiccups.

✓ Dissolve a tablespoon of organic honey in a warm glass of water and sip it slowly.

✓ Chew three slices of fresh ginger and slowly swallow it. This is an ancient Chinese method for coping with hiccups. If it doesn't work, complain to the ancient Chinese.

✓ Put in earplugs and slowly sip a glass of warm or cold water.

✓ Place half a teaspoon of whole mustard seeds in your mouth, chew, and swallow.

✓ Measure out a half teaspoon of salt. Take up small amounts with your tongue and slowly swallow it.

✓ Inhale. Hold your breath as long as you can.

✓ Breathe into a paper bag grasped tightly around your mouth for a few minutes.

✓ Acupressure: Place your middle and index fingers behind each earlobe. Apply light to firm pressure on these tender points for 2 minutes as you concentrate on breathing slowly and deeply.

And Try This!

Try melting a teaspoonful of sugar on your tongue. Long considered good for nothing nutritionally, apparently sugar is good for something—hiccups—says Edgar E. Engleman, M.D., of the University of California School of Medicine in San Francisco. Dr. Engleman tried it on 20 patients, and it stopped hiccups in 19 cases.

Did You Know?

A farmer named Charles Osborne—believe it or not—hiccuped for 60 years. He wasn't trying to get into the *Guinness Book of World Records*. He just couldn't find a remedy that worked.

High Blood Pressure (Hypertension)

High blood pressure increases the risk of dying due to heart attack by 52 percent and of congestive heart failure by 63 percent. If that doesn't get your attention, nothing will. Except maybe for the fact that 1 out of every 4 Americans suffers from it to some degree. Still not concerned? How about the knowledge that it is rarely accompanied by noticeable symptoms, hence its nickname—The Silent Killer!

Recognizing High Blood Pressure

The force that blood exerts on your arteries and veins is represented by two figures: systolic, the degree of force exerted when the heart is beating, and diastolic, the degree of force exerted when the heart is resting. Normal blood pressure is represented by 120 (systolic) over 80 (diastolic)—or lower. Mild hypertension is usually defined by 140 over 90 or more. Extreme high blood pressure drives the numbers off the chart. The worst place to get an accurate reading on blood pressure is the doctor's office. "White coat" syndrome causes blood pressure to register far higher than it is. Two readings should be taken—one twenty minutes after arrival there and then just before leaving. However, best results come from testing yourself at home with a blood pressure measuring device (sphygmomanometer).

What Are the Causes of High Blood Pressure?

High blood pressure is generally classified medically as either *primary* or *secondary hypertension,* depending on the cause. In patients diagnosed with secondary hypertension, the source of their high blood pressure is a recognizable illness, often arteriosclerosis or kidney trouble. Primary hypertension is that which is not the result of an underlying illness and where no direct cause has been identified. Over 90 percent of Americans diagnosed with high blood pressure fall into this category. Known risk factors for primary hypertension include the following:

- Family history
- Smoking
- Stress
- Caffeine (especially in coffee)
- Alcohol
- Drug use
- Birth control pills
- Diet high in sugar and other refined carbohydrates
- Diet high in salt
- Lack of exercise
- Overweight
- Crash diets
- Nutritional deficiencies
- High levels of the heavy metal cadmium in the body

What You Can Take

Nutrients

Name	Dosage	Benefits
Vitamin C	500 mg three times daily	Opens blood vessels wider and contributes to their strength and integrity.
Calcium	1,000 mg daily	Can significantly lower high blood pressure.
Coenzyme Q-10	50 mg twice daily	Helps lower elevated blood pressure and corrects other cardiovascular conditions.
Magnesium	500 mg daily	Deficiencies linked to high blood pressure and poor circulation. Supplements can return blood pressure to normal.
Omega-3 essential fatty acids	1,000 mg softgel three times daily	Rich in essential fatty acids that improve blood circulation and protect against high blood pressure.
Potassium	100 mg daily	Reduces the risk of high blood pressure as well as stroke.
Taurine	500 mg between meals	Removes excess body fluid, which helps to lower blood pressure.

Name	Dosage	Benefits
Arginine	1,000 mg between meals *Warning:* Do not take if you have kidney disease, genital herpes, or repeated cold sores.	Plays a key role in synthesizing nitric oxide, which relaxes artery walls for more free blood flow.
Zinc chelate	15–30 mg daily	Protects against high blood pressure indirectly by blocking the body's accumulation of the heavy metal cadmium.

Herbs

Name	Dosage	Benefits
Garlic (odorless)	400–1,200 mg daily	All-purpose aid for various cardiovascular disorders. Blocks blood fats from sticking to the interior of arteries and reducing blood circulation.

What You Can Do

✓ Have your blood pressure checked at least twice a year.
✓ Don't smoke.
✓ Avoid alcohol and caffeine.
✓ Avoid sugar and other refined carbohydrates.
✓ Limit your intake of salt.
✓ Exercise regularly.
✓ Drink at least 8–10 glasses of pure spring water daily.
✓ Maintain healthy body weight (*see* OVERWEIGHT).
✓ Work to relieve stress (*see* STRESS).
✓ Avoid antihistamines unless taken under the supervision of your doctor.
✓ Add a serving of fresh fruits and vegetables to every meal.
✓ Eat foods high in vitamin C, including rose hips, acerola cherries, guavas, black currants, red peppers, oranges, grape-

fruit and other citrus fruits, cabbage, papayas, cantaloupe, and tomatoes.

✓ Eat foods high in calcium, including buttermilk, milk, yogurt, cheddar, parmesan and romano cheese, carob, brewer's yeast, broccoli, kale, kelp, amaranth, teff, almonds and sesame seeds.

✓ Eat foods high in coenzyme Q-10, including salmon, sardines, mackerel, and spinach.

✓ Eat foods high in magnesium, including blackstrap molasses, sunflower seeds, wheat germ, almonds, hazelnuts, Brazil nuts, pecans, walnuts, soybeans, soy lecithin, oats, barley, salmon, corn, avocados, bananas, cheese, tuna, and potatoes.

✓ Eat foods high in potassium, including bananas, cantaloupe, broccoli, avocados, Brussels sprouts, cauliflower, blackstrap molasses, brewer's yeast, brown rice, potatoes, legumes, dates, and whole grains.

✓ Eat foods high in zinc, including seafood, sardines, oysters, soybeans, soy lecithin, kelp, legumes, meat, liver, eggs, brewer's yeast, mushrooms, poultry, whole grains, and pumpkin and sunflower seeds.

And Try This!

Try drinking a cup of hawthorn tea twice daily. It is known for dilating and relaxing arteries throughout the body, thus lowering blood pressure. Do not use, however, if you are taking digitalis medications.

Did You Know?

Although some evidence indicates that one glass of wine daily can contribute to normal blood pressure, most studies reveal that even moderate alcohol drinking increases blood pressure by stimulating secretion of stress hormones from the adrenal glands.

High Cholesterol

After years of warnings against the evils of high cholesterol as
it pertains to increased risks for heart disease, stroke, and other
life-threatening ailments, the momentum is shifting from lowering blood cholesterol levels in general to assuring a healthy
balance between the two different types of cholesterol: low-
density lipoproteins (LDL) and high-density lipoproteins (HDL).
Most of the cholesterol required by the body is produced in the
liver. Low-density lipoproteins are responsible for carrying this
cholesterol from the liver to all the other cells throughout the
body. It is then the job of high-density lipoproteins to collect
the leftover cholesterol and return it to the liver, where it can be
transported out to the cells again when needed. Trouble occurs
when there are not enough high-density lipoproteins to retrieve
all the excess cholesterol, allowing it to build up as plaque in
the arteries.

Recognizing High Cholesterol

Cholesterol levels should be checked regularly by your doctor, preferably as part of an annual physical exam. You will re-
ceive a reading for total cholesterol and individual readings for
both LDL (bad cholesterol) and HDL (good cholesterol). Total
cholesterol readings above 230 mg/dl are considered high risk,
as are LDL levels above 159 mg/dl and HDL levels below 35
mg/dl. But more important is the ratio between your total cholesterol level and that of your HDL. A 4:1 ratio or lower is ideal.
A ratio of 5:1 or higher is reason for concern.

What Are the Causes of High Cholesterol?

- Family history
- High-cholesterol, high-fat diet
- Lack of exercise
- Stress
- Smoking

What You Can Take

Nutrients

Name	Dosage	Benefits
Vitamin C	1,000 mg daily	Proven cholesterol-lowering effects.

What You Can Do

- ✓ Exercise daily.
- ✓ Drink at least 8–10 glasses of pure spring water daily.
- ✓ Avoid alcohol and coffee.
- ✓ Avoid sugar and other refined carbohydrates.
- ✓ Don't smoke.
- ✓ Maintain a healthy body weight (*see* OVERWEIGHT).
- ✓ Relieve stress (*see* STRESS).
- ✓ Eat foods that studies have shown can help lower cholesterol, including apples, avocados, barley, beans, carrots, chili pepper, eggplant, garlic, grapefruit, red grapes, skim milk, oats, olive oil, onions, plantains, seafood, seaweed (kelp), soy (in the form of lecithin, soy milk, and tofu), spinach, yams, and yogurt.
- ✓ Be aware that conventional cholesterol-lowering drugs often have serious side effects. Do not begin taking any such medications before a thorough review of the potential side effects with your doctor.

And Try This!

Try eating five or six small meals throughout the day as opposed to the standard three square meals. Heavy meals make the pancreas release large amounts of insulin. This triggers the production of an enzyme that revs up the production of cholesterol by the liver.

Did You Know?

Biochemist Joseph Patsch, of Baylor College of Medicine, had volunteers do fast walking or jogging for 20–25 minutes daily. Soon their serum cholesterol and blood fat levels dropped steadily, as HDL increased in ratio to LDL.

Hives

Hives are raised, swollen, red skin blotches with white centers that can itch a person to distraction. Hives may vary in size and appear on any area of the body, but are most common on the arms and legs. Generally brought about by an allergic reaction, you almost need a scorecard to identify all the things that can trigger hives.

Recognizing Hives

- Skin rash that appears suddenly and may spread
- Rash takes the form of raised red blotches with white centers
- Appearance of wheals or welts that can resemble insect bites
- Itching and swelling

What Are the Causes of Hives?

- Food and environmental allergies are the primary causes of hives. And the list of triggers is almost endless. The following are just some of the most widely recognized examples: beans, soy, eggs, fish, shellfish, meat, dairy products, poultry, nuts, wheat, sugar, raisins, prunes, strawberries, grapes, dried apricots, soft drinks, alcohol, food additives, food colorings, food preservatives, penicillin, antibiotics, aspirin, fluoride, pesticides, household cleaners, and mercury
- Stress
- Viral or bacterial infections (especially hepatitis B)
- Yeast overgrowth

What You Can Take

Nutrients

Name	Dosage	Benefits
Vitamin B$_{12}$	1 mg intravenously or 1,000 mcg under the tongue three times daily	Helpful against both acute and chronic cases of hives.
Vitamin C	1,000 mg three times daily	Natural antihistamine that has been shown to benefit patients with hives.
Quercetin	200–400 mg three times daily, a half hour before meals	Blocks the release of histamine and keeps histamine from being formed.

What You Can Do

- ✓ Test for food and environmental allergies (*see* ALLERGIES).
- ✓ Avoid processed foods, which are loaded with additives, colorings, and preservatives.
- ✓ Work to relieve stress (*see* STRESS).
- ✓ Apply aloe vera gel to hives to relieve pain and itching.
- ✓ Eat foods high in vitamin B$_{12}$, including liver, sardines, mackerel, herring, red snapper, flounder, salmon, lamb, Swiss cheese, blue cheese, eggs, haddock, beef, halibut, anchovies, chicken, turkey, milk, and butter.
- ✓ Eat foods high in vitamin C, including rose hips, acerola cherries, guavas, black currants, red peppers, oranges, grapefruit and other citrus fruits, cabbage, papayas, cantaloupe, and tomatoes.

And Try This!

Try paying very close attention to everything you may have eaten or been exposed to prior to the onset of hives. It may sound obvious, but hives can appear suddenly when exposed to an allergen. A little detective work can go a long way toward preventing them in the future!

Did You Know?

According to a study published in the *British Medical Journal*, twice as many patients with hives responded positively to a yeast-free diet—no beer, bread, buns, cider, grapes, pickles, vinegar, and processed foods containing yeast—as to 3 weeks on the prescription drug nystatin.

Hyperthyroidism

Remember how your motor races and your car vibrates when you floor the accelerator? Something similar happens in your body when you produce too much thyroid hormone. Your heart beats in high gear, your blood volume increases, and your blood pressure soars. You become overheated, perspire freely, your hands shake, and you feel so jittery that you almost want to leap out of your skin. However, when thyroid hormone secretion is just slightly excessive, patients often are superenergetic, self-assured, enthusiastic, and optimistic. This state is not unlike a mild manic phase of manic depression. Usually the condition worsens, so the person eventually must see a doctor for diagnosis and treatment.

Recognizing Hyperthyroidism

Hyperthyroidism is far rarer than hypothyroidism (its opposite), which leads some doctors to treat a major symptom of the disorder and fail to test for abnormal thyroid function. It is important to request such tests at the first warning signs of hyperthyroidism:

- High, sometimes manic energy states
- Irregular heartbeats
- High blood pressure
- Sweating
- Shaking hands
- Anxiety
- Panic attacks
- Irritability
- Bulging eyes

Symptoms can become more extreme if the condition is left untreated, and may then include the following:

- Hair loss
- Heart muscle damage
- Kidney damage
- Stroke
- Excessive amounts of bone calcium loss
- Diminished sense of reality
- Paranoia
- Hallucinations
- Visual and auditory delusions

What Are the Causes of Hyperthyroidism?

Hyperthyroidism is the result of the thyroid gland producing too much thyroid hormone. Contributing factors are believed to include:

- Family history
- Nutritional deficiencies
- Underlying illness
- Weak immune system that mistakenly attacks the thyroid gland

What You Can Take

Nutrients

Name	Dosage	Benefits
Vitamin B-complex	100 mg daily	Contains vitamins B_1 and B_6, both of which are rapidly burned up and depleted by hyperthyroid.
Vitamin C	500 mg three times daily	Deficiencies can cause the thyroid gland to bleed, multiply normal cells abnormally, and secrete too much thyroid hormone.
Vitamin D	400 IU daily	Slows down the rapid excretion of calcium in hyperthyroid, protecting the integrity of bones.
Vitamin E	400 IU daily	Deficiencies can cause the thyroid gland to multiply normal cells abnormally and se-

Name	Dosage	Benefits
		crete too much thyroid hormone.
Multivitamin and mineral complex	As directed on label	Protects against wide-scale deficiencies that can result from hyperthyroidism.
Magnesium	500 mg daily	Deficiencies linked to hyperthyroidism.
Evening primrose oil	Two 500 mg capsules three times daily	High in essential fatty acids, deficiencies of which have been linked to hyperthyroidism.
Borage oil	1,000 mg daily	High in essential fatty acids, deficiencies of which have been linked to hyperthyroidism.
Black currant seed oil	1,500 mg daily	High in essential fatty acids, deficiencies of which have been linked to hyperthyroidism.

What You Can Do

✓ Be tested by a doctor if you suspect you may be hyperthyroid.
✓ Avoid caffeine.
✓ Don't smoke.
✓ Eat thyroid-suppressing foods, including cabbage, cauliflower, broccoli, Brussels sprouts, kale, mustard greens, peaches, rutabagas, spinach, and turnips.
✓ Eat foods high in calcium, including buttermilk, milk, yogurt (lowfat), cheddar, parmesan and romano cheese, carob, brewer's yeast, broccoli, kale, kelp, amaranth, teff, almonds and sesame seeds.
✓ Eat foods high in vitamin C, including rose hips, acerola cherries, guavas, black currants, red peppers, oranges, grapefruit and other citrus fruits, cabbage, papayas, cantaloupe, and tomatoes.
✓ Eat foods high in vitamin E, including sunflower seeds, whole

wheat, peanuts, cashews, almonds, walnuts, corn oil, soy oil, soy lecithin, spinach, asparagus, broccoli, butter oats, and avocados.

✓ Eat foods high in magnesium, including blackstrap molasses, sunflower seeds, wheat germ, almonds, hazelnuts, Brazil nuts, pecans, walnuts, soybeans, soy lecithin, oats, barley, salmon, corn, avocados, bananas, cheese, tuna, and potatoes.

✓ Eat foods high in vitamin D, including cod liver oil, eggs, herring, organ meats, salmon, and sardines.

And Try This!

Some doctors prescribe thyroid hormone for managing this condition, even though the problem is excessive secretion of this hormone. Why? Additional thyroid hormone in the bloodstream signals the pituitary gland to stop producing thyroid-stimulating hormone, so this shuts down production by the thyroid gland, usually reducing the secretion to normal.

Did You Know?

Conventional medicine calls for destroying or at least inactivating thyroid tissue to slow down the secretion of thyroid hormones in one of three ways: by means of antithyroid drugs, radioactive iodine, or surgery. Each of these poses danger if not handled sensitively—shutting off hormone production entirely, causing low thyroid function, and triggering many side effects. Don't be stampeded into such treatments of the thyroid gland. Get a second opinion, or a third if necessary, preferably from a physician familiar with the natural approaches discussed here.

Hypoglycemia (Low Blood Sugar)

One of the great imitators among human ailments is hypoglycemia, low blood sugar. It has at least forty symptoms typical of other disorders. However, the first thing you should understand about hypoglycemia is how, unknowingly, you may be cooperating with this enemy within to undermine your energy and your life's objectives.

Recognizing Hypoglycemia

Energy surges followed by tiredness after the eating of refined carbohydrates or the drinking of coffee is the most revealing symptom of hypoglycemia. However, there are many others. Exhaustion, nervousness, and irritability are also top symptoms manifested by hypoglycemic patients. They are most common in the late afternoon. Additional symptoms may include:

- Faintness
- Depression
- Dizziness
- Drowsiness
- Headaches
- Digestive disorders
- Forgetfulness
- Sleeplessness
- Constant worrying
- Mental confusion
- Irregular heartbeat
- Muscle pain
- Excessive hunger (especially for sweets)

What Are the Causes of Hypoglycemia?

Hypoglycemia results from the way that your body handles or mishandles sugar, rather than just the amount of sugar in the bloodstream at any particular time. This is primarily due to the pancreas secreting too much insulin. Contributing factors can include:

- Diet high in sugar and other refined carbohydrates
- Diet low in complex carbohydrates
- Skipping meals (especially breakfast)
- Nutritional deficiencies (especially chromium)
- Food allergies
- Low thyroid function
- Stress
- Alcohol
- Caffeine
- Smoking
- Poor digestion
- Family history
- Diabetes
- Adrenal exhaustion
- Yeast overgrowth

What You Can Take

Nutrients

Name	Dosage	Benefits
Vitamin B-complex	100 mg daily	Deficiencies can result in hypoglycemia.
Alpha-lipoic acid	600 mg daily	Stabilizes blood sugar levels.
Chromium	200 mcg daily	Lowers blood sugar levels by improving the efficiency of insulin.
Vanadyl sulfate	20–40 mg daily	Enhances the proper functioning of insulin, helping to normalize hypoglycemic symptoms.

Herbs

Name	Dosage	Benefits
Gymnema sylvestre	400 mg daily	Stabilizes blood sugar levels.

What You Can Do

✓ Avoid the following foods: sugar, corn syrup (in many processed foods), candies, cake, pastries, pies, dates, raisins, figs, prunes, bananas, corn, sweet potatoes, sweet cherries, beans (kidney, lima, and navy), macaroni, spaghetti, white rice, sweetened soft drinks, processed cereals, coffee (and all other forms of caffeine), and alcohol.

✓ Eat the following foods sparingly: apples, apricots, blueberries, sour cherries, currants, grapes, huckleberries, loganberries, nectarines, pears, pineapples, plums, artichokes, parsnips, peas, cantaloupe, oranges, peaches, fresh raspberries, hubbard squash, and turnips.

✓ Eat the following foods regularly: fresh string beans, carrots, cauliflower, okra, onions, peppers, pumpkin, avocado, radishes, lettuce, watercress, beef, lamb, poultry, fish, cheese, and milk (if you're not milk intolerant or allergic).

✓ Eat five or six small meals a day with the same number of calories as the three customarily eaten.

✓ Never skip meals (especially breakfast).
✓ Don't smoke.
✓ Exercise daily.
✓ Relieve stress (*see* STRESS).
✓ Test for low thyroid (*see* HYPOTHYROIDISM).
✓ Test for food allergies (*see* ALLERGIES).

And Try This!

If nothing else works, try a little known way of dealing with hypoglycemia—supplementing with magnesium. Four hundred milligrams of this mineral have helped some of my patients eliminate this condition.

Did You Know?

A double-blind, crossover study published in the journal *Metabolism* reported that patients experienced significant corrections in their hypoglycemic symptoms after taking 200 mcg of chromium chloride twice daily for 3 months.

Hypothyroidism (Low Thyroid Function)

Hypothyroidism is a common condition in the United States. Conservative estimates indicate it affects more than 5 million people, nine out of every ten of them being women. Many experts argue the numbers are much higher, and that most of those suffering from low thyroid function remain undiagnosed.

The thyroid gland regulates the metabolism in every one of our trillions of cells. It is essential to developing energy and body warmth. Consider this analogy as to how it works: the efficient burning of a fire made with dry wood is normal thyroid function, whereas the incomplete combustion of a fire made with wet wood—along with the resulting smoke and sputtering—is subnormal thyroid function with too little hormone.

Recognizing Hypothyroidism

Numerous studies reveal that as many as 64 symptoms can originate from low thyroid function. The most telltale are deep fatigue—the depression that accompanies fatigue—and icy hands and feet and feeling cold while others in the room are comfortable. Additional symptoms may include the following:

- High cholesterol levels
- Arteriosclerosis
- Weak heartbeat
- Heart palpitations
- Dry, coarse, and pale skin
- Lethargy
- Slow speech
- Swelling of face and eyelids
- Pale skin
- Constipation
- Fertility problems
- Menstrual disorders
- Diminished sexual desire
- Thick tongue
- Weight gain
- Hair loss
- Labored breathing
- Swollen feet
- Hoarseness
- Nervousness
- Brittle nails
- Headaches
- Slow movement
- Difficulty in thinking and remembering
- Emotional instability
- Depression
- Frequent colds and other upper respiratory infections

If you suspect you may be hypothyroid based on this list, take the *Barnes Basal Temperature Test*—a do-it-yourself means of checking thyroid gland function. The test was developed by Dr. Broda O. Barnes, a world authority on thyroid gland function. It works like this:

Immediately after you wake up from a good night's sleep (not a minute later) tuck a thermometer smugly in your armpit for 10 minutes as you lie still. If your thyroid function is normal, your temperature should range from 97.8 to 98.2 degrees F (women get the most accurate results when not menstruating or on the second and third days of menstruation). If the temperature registers less, you may be hypothyroid. Take this test for two consecutive days, and see a physician for further testing if results are less than 97.8 degree both times.

What Are the Causes of Hypothyroidism?

Hypothyroidism results mainly from a failure of the thyroid gland to produce enough thyroid hormone. Contributing factors are believed to include:

- Family history
- Insufficient iodine intake (only an infinitesimal amount is required)
- Thyroid gland inhibitors in foods and beverages
- Nutritional deficiencies
- Hashimoto's disease, a condition in which the body becomes allergic to the thyroid gland and produces antibodies against it

What You Can Take

Nutrients

Name	Dosage	Benefits
Vitamin A	10,000 IU daily	Contributes to secretion of thyroid hormone. Deficiencies linked to hypothyroidism.
Vitamin B-complex	100 mg daily	Vitamins B_2, B_6, B_{12}, and niacin are essential to the secretion of thyroid hormone. Deficiencies of these B vitamins have been linked to hypothyroidism.
Vitamin C	500 mg three times daily	Keeps thyroid gland healthy so it can work properly. Deficiencies linked to hypothyroidism.
Vitamin E	400 IU daily	A *must* for the pituitary gland to know when to turn on thyroid hormone production. Deficiencies linked to hypothyroidism.
Armour natural desiccated thyroid hormone	As prescribed by physician	Compensates for the inability of the thyroid gland to secrete enough hormone.

What You Can Do

✓ Take the Barnes Basal Temperature Test.
✓ Drink at least 8–10 glasses of pure spring water daily.
✓ Avoid fluoridated water (fluoride is a known thyroid suppressant).
✓ Avoid sulfa drugs and antihistamines (which limit thyroid hormone production).
✓ Avoid thyroid-suppressing foods, including cabbage, cauliflower, broccoli, Brussels sprouts, kale, mustard greens, peaches, rutabagas, spinach, and turnips.
✓ Eat foods high in vitamin A, including eggs, milk, cheese, cream, butter, yogurt, salmon, bass, halibut, mackerel, herring, whitefish, sardines, tuna, clams, shrimp, beef, chicken, pistachios, pecans, walnuts, lentils, and soybeans.
✓ Eat foods high in vitamin B_2, including brewer's yeast, alfalfa, liver, royal jelly, bee pollen, almonds, wheat germ, egg yolk, cheese, millet, chicken, mushrooms, soybeans, sunflower seeds, lamb, peas, blackstrap molasses, cottage cheese, sesame seeds, lentils, whole rye, and turkey.
✓ Eat foods high in vitamin B_6, including brewer's yeast, brown rice, whole wheat, royal jelly, soybeans, whole rye, lentils, sunflower seeds, alfalfa, salmon, wheat germ, tuna, bran, walnuts, cashews, peanuts, peas, liver, avocados, beans, turkey, oats, chicken, halibut, lamb, and bananas.
✓ Eat foods high in vitamin B_{12}, including liver, sardines, mackerel, herring, red snapper, flounder, salmon, lamb, Swiss cheese, blue cheese, eggs, haddock, beef, halibut, scallops, anchovies, chicken, turkey, milk, and butter.
✓ Eat foods high in vitamin C, including rose hips, acerola cherries, guavas, black currants, red peppers, oranges, grapefruit and other citrus fruits, papayas, cantaloupe, kiwi fruit, and tomatoes.
✓ Eat foods high in vitamin E, including whole wheat, wheat germ, wheat germ oil, olive oil, butter, safflower seeds, sunflower seeds, peanuts, cashews, almonds, walnuts, hazelnuts, soy lecithin, asparagus, oats, and avocados.

And Try This!

If synthetic thyroid hormones have not helped, try Armour desiccated natural thyroid. Research has shown that synthetics containing only the T4 fraction do not always convert to T3 (the body-active hormone) in the human body. Natural thyroid, on the other hand, contains T4, T3 and T2 and has been found to compensate for hypothyroidism most efficiently.

Did You Know?

Two thousand years before Christ, Chinese doctors revived energy and rejuvenated failing patients by feeding them an animal thyroid soup. During the late nineteenth century and early twentieth century—before there were thyroid pills—London's most prominent Harley Street physicians helped revive weak and rapidly aging patients with a raw animal thyroid in sandwiches. This was the forerunner to glandulars sold in health food stores.

Impotence

One of the blackest days or nights in a man's life is marked by failure in the bedroom. Panic is the first time you can't do it the second time. Disaster is the second time you can't do it the first time. Where to turn? To the friendly neighborhood urologist—preferably an alternative or complementary physician. The latter uses conventional and unconventional methods to get a man functioning again.

Recognizing Impotence

Recognize it? Are you kidding! Just ask one of the approximately 30 million American men who have, at least on occasion, suffered from impotence to come up with a list of symptoms. A short list indeed—the failure to achieve or sustain an erection at a level required for sexual intercourse.

What Are the Causes of Impotence?

Contrary to what you may believe, experts agree that the majority of impotence cases are physiological rather than psychological in origin. The best way to tell is if you achieve erections in your sleep. If so, the problem most likely involves emotional issues that may be best addressed by a professional counselor. In cases that are physiological in nature, the problem is generally that of restricted blood flow to the penis. Contributing factors may include:

- Smoking
- Alcohol
- Diabetes
- Impaired blood circulation
- High blood pressure
- Prescription medications
- History of sexually transmitted disease

What You Can Take

Nutrients

Name	Dosage	Benefits
Vitamin B-complex	100 mg daily	Exerts a powerful influence on the secretion of testosterone, the male hormone essential to sexual desire and erections.
Vitamin C	1,000 mg three times daily	Enhances blood circulation.
Ginkgo biloba	80 mg daily	Dilates capillaries and enhances blood circulation.
L-arginine	1–2 g daily *Warning:* Do not take if you have kidney disease, genital herpes, or repeated cold sores.	Contributes to renewed sexual ability and increased sperm count.
Zinc	30 mg daily	Important to the secretion of testosterone, the male hormone essential to sexual desire and erections.

Herbs

Name	Dosage	Benefits
Yohimbe	15–30 mg twice daily	Used for centuries as an aphrodisiac and treatment for impotence.

What You Can Do

✓ Keep trying!
✓ Don't smoke.
✓ Avoid alcohol.
✓ Avoid sugar and other refined carbohydrates.
✓ Exercise regularly.
✓ Relieve stress (*see* STRESS).
✓ Discuss with your physician potential side effects of any medication you may believe could be causing the problem with your physician.
✓ Eat foods high in vitamin C, including rose hips, acerola cherries, guavas, black currants, red peppers, oranges, grapefruit and other citrus fruits, cabbage, papayas, cantaloupe, and tomatoes.
✓ Eat foods high in zinc, including seafood, sardines, oysters, soybeans, soy lecithin, kelp, legumes, meat, liver, eggs, brewer's yeast, mushrooms, poultry, whole grains, and pumpkin and sunflower seeds.
✓ Test (hair analysis) for toxic levels of heavy metals such as mercury in the body.
✓ Consider chelation therapy, a safe and effective means of ridding the body of heavy metals. Chelation therapy can be performed either orally or intravenously and has been used successfully to improve blood circulation. Please consult with a physician trained in this practice, as it requires close medical supervision.

And Try This!

Try drinking muira puama tea—a teaspoonful per cup in the morning and at noon. A Brazilian herb, muira puama is best known in Great Britain for alleviating impotence, and as an aphrodisiac.

Did You Know?

Some years ago two Canadian doctors tested yohimbe on 23 impotent men. Ten improved, and six gained full sexual function. Soon after these men quit taking yohimbe, their potency declined. Then Stanford University researchers tested this substance on rats and got similar results. Rats demonstrated heightened sexual response, and the researchers concluded that yohimbe works by increasing the effects of the hormone norepinephrine in the brain's pleasure center.

Incontinence (Involuntary Urinating)

"It's awful, Doctor! I'm middle-aged and back where I started fifty years ago—in diapers!" Deanna was not only incontinent—unable to control urine leakage and, therefore, wearing a protective, padded undergarment—but angry and at a loss for what to do. Deanna is also not alone. Few conditions cause as much embarrassment and go so untalked about as incontinence.

Recognizing Incontinence

There are four major kinds of incontinence: stress, urge, total, and overflow.

Stress incontinence occurs when a person coughs, sneezes, laughs, exercises, or strains when constipated. Small amounts of urine dribble out. This is not uncommon—particularly following childbirth, which causes stretching of sphincter muscles, ringlike muscles that control closing and opening of the urethra, the passage for discharging urine.

Urge incontinence often comes on so suddenly that it's impossible to make it to a restroom.

Total incontinence is complete loss of bladder control because the sphincter fails.

Overflow incontinence is the inability to drain the bladder fully because of a blockage, with occasional leakage of small amounts of urine from the overflow. However, surgery that removes the blockage usually renews continence.

What Are the Causes of Incontinence?

- Urinary tract infections
- Flabby and weak muscles
- Hormonal problems
- Neurological ailments
- Overweight
- Lack of physical activity
- Alcohol
- Caffeine
- Diet high in sugar and other refined carbohydrates
- Smoking

What You Can Take

Nutrients

Name	Dosage	Benefits
Magnesium	300 mg twice daily	Minimizes incontinence.

Herbs

Name	Dosage	Benefits
Echinacea	200 mg six times daily for infections	Helps fight urinary tract infections, a common cause of incontinence.
Garlic (odorless)	Two 300 mg capsules three times daily	Helps fight urinary tract infections, a common cause of incontinence.
St. John's wort	300 mg three times daily	Shown positive results in the treatment of incontinence.

What You Can Do

✓ Drink at least 8-10 glasses of pure spring water daily.
✓ Eat plenty of fresh raw fruits and vegetables.
✓ Don't smoke.
✓ Avoid alcohol and caffeine.
✓ Avoid sugar and other refined carbohydrates.
✓ Avoid processed foods.
✓ Exercise regularly.
✓ Maintain ideal body weight (*see* OVERWEIGHT).
✓ Avoid recurring urinary tract infections (*see* CYSTITIS).

And Try This!

Try the Kegel method for coping with incontinence. A simple exercise, it involves tightening the muscles that stop urine flow and holding them for a count of 10, then urinating slowly, stopping again and repeating the routine until the bladder is empty. This should be done 8-10 times daily. Muscle tone starts improving within 10 days to 2 weeks and, with it, better control of flow.

Did You Know?

Writing in the *Townsend Letter for Doctors & Patients,* Dr. Alan R. Gaby of Seattle reported on a double-blind study of 40 middle-age women with symptoms of incontinence. Subjects received either 300 mg of magnesium hydroxide twice daily for 4 weeks or a placebo. When no improvement was noted within 2 weeks, the researchers doubled their magnesium intake for the next 2 weeks. Results indicated that 55 percent of those who took magnesium experienced relief compared to just 20 percent of the placebo takers.

Infertility/Sterility (Male)

Estimates are that 20 percent or more of American couples experience issues of infertility at some point in their relationship. Once upon a time the woman was always blamed if she couldn't become pregnant. Biochemical researchers now find that it's a 50–50 proposition between the sexes.

Recognizing Infertility/Sterility

A couple is generally recognized as experiencing signs of infertility if they are unable to conceive after a year of actively trying through regular sexual intercourse. At this point, tests are conducted to identify which partner is the likely source of the problem.

What Are the Causes of Infertility/Sterility?

In men suffering from infertility, the trouble is in the sperm cells. There may be too few of them (sperm count). They may not be active enough (sperm motility). Or they may stick together (sperm agglutination). Factors that contribute to these conditions can include the following:

- Smoking
- Alcohol
- Caffeine
- Injury to the testicles
- Testicles exposed to excessive heat
- Anatomical disorders
- Prescription medications
- Nutritional deficiencies

What You Can Take

Nutrients

Name	Dosage	Benefits
Vitamin B-complex	100 mg daily	Vitamin B_{12} raises sperm count. Deficiencies are linked to low sperm counts.
Vitamin C	500 mg daily	Corrects sperm clumping and increases sperm count.

Name	Dosage	Benefits
Vitamin E	100–200 IU daily	Assists the development of healthy and superactive sperm.
Coenzyme Q-10	10 mg daily	Increases sperm count and sperm motility.
Ginkgo biloba	60 mg three times daily	Increases blood circulation, circulating oxygen, nutrients and thyroid hormone to areas where sperm cells are made.
L-arginine	1,000 mg twice daily *Warning:* Do not take if you have kidney disease, genital herpes, or repeated cold sores.	Increases sperm count and sperm motility.
L-carnitine	500 mg twice daily	Increases sperm count and sperm motility.
Zinc	120 mg of zinc sulfate daily for 40–50 days *Warning:* This amount should be accompanied by 2 mg of copper to maintain proper ratio.	Raises testosterone and sperm count.

What You Can Do

✓ Exercise regularly.
✓ Don't smoke.
✓ Avoid alcohol and caffeine.
✓ Limit exposure of testicles to excessive heat such as hot baths.
✓ Consult with physician concerning side effects to any prescription drugs you may be taking.
✓ Eat plenty of fresh fruits, vegetables, and whole grains.
✓ Eat foods high in vitamin B_{12}, including liver, sardines, mackerel, herring, red snapper, flounder, salmon, lamb, Swiss cheese, blue cheese, eggs, haddock, beef, halibut, anchovies, chicken, turkey, milk, and butter.
✓ Eat foods high in vitamin C, including rose hips, acerola

cherries, guavas, black currants, red peppers, oranges, grapefruit and other citrus fruits, cabbage, papayas, cantaloupe, and tomatoes.

✓ Eat foods high in vitamin E, including sunflower seeds, whole wheat, peanuts, cashews, almonds, walnuts, corn oil, soy oil, soy lecithin, spinach, asparagus, broccoli, oats, and avocados.

✓ Eat foods high in zinc, including seafood, sardines, oysters, soybeans, soy lecithin, kelp, legumes, meat, liver, eggs, brewer's yeast, mushrooms, poultry, whole grains, and pumpkin and sunflower seeds.

And Try This!

If your sperm has not made your mate pregnant, try supplementing with aged, odorless garlic. Several urologists have told me that 400 mg of garlic supplement three times daily has upgraded the sperm counts of their patients to their proper levels.

Did You Know?

A study by Dr. Earl B. Dawson, at the University of Texas Medical Branch, involved 35 men with a 20 percent sperm agglutination rate with marginal blood levels of vitamin C. Supplemented with 500 mg of vitamin C for 3 weeks, they showed a drop of 11 percent in their sperm agglutination rate. Twelve of the men were able to make their wives pregnant. Over and above a sharp decline of sperm agglutination, men on this regimen for 60 days revealed more sperm of greater quality and highly active.

Insect Bites

In his classic *Archy and Mehitabel*, Don Marquis put things in proper perspective: "... a man thinks he amounts to a great deal, but to the flea or mosquito, a human being is merely something good to eat." True! So our best defensive strategy is to make ourselves less appetizing. But defense against insects is only half the story. Coping with bites and stings is the other. Thankfully, there are natural ways to do both.

Recognizing Insect Bites

- Localized redness or itching of the skin
- Sudden poking or pinching pain
- Throbbing or burning pain
- Fever, breathing difficulties, confusion, general weakness (in case of allergic reactions to bee stings)

What Are the Causes of Insect Bites?

Insects have to eat!

What You Can Take

Nutrients

Name	Dosage	Benefits
Vitamin B-complex	100 mg daily	Repels mosquitoes and some other insects.

Herbs

Name	Dosage	Benefits
Garlic	Two 600 mg capsules daily	Works as a repellant to many insects.
Blue or black cohosh	Two to three 40 mg capsules daily	Repels mosquitoes.

What You Can Do

✓ Make yourself unattractive to insects by eating a daily clove of garlic.
✓ Avoid alcohol and sugar. (Insects like it, too!)
✓ Add a teaspoonful of brewer's yeast to a glass of spring water or tomato juice and drink daily.

✓ Apply the following mixture to heal insect bites: a capsule of goldenseal powder mixed in a tablespoon of aloe vera juice.

✓ Aloe vera gel alone is also effective when applied to insect bites and bee stings in soothing, speeding healing, and preventing scars.

✓ Scrape away a bee stinger, wash the affected area with soap and water, and apply the goldenseal–aloe vera mix frequently.

✓ Shake one capsule of plantain powder on bee stings or mix it with 1 tablespoon of aloe vera and spread it on.

✓ Apply tea tree oil to bites (it is a disinfectant, an antibiotic, and a fungicide).

✓ Spread calendula ointment, an antiseptic and astringent, on insect bites.

✓ Fasten freshly cut onion slices on insect bites to prevent infection and promote fast healing.

And Try This!

Try making a paste of Adolph's meat tenderizer and water and apply it immediately to insect bites to reduce swelling and aid healing. I'm not putting you on. It really works!

Did You Know?

Sardinians ward off mosquitoes by rubbing garlic juice on all exposed parts of their bodies. And Sardinian mosquitoes avoid garlic for more than just its odor. Contact with it kills them. Presumably, mosquitoes worldwide are also bright enough to avoid garlic.

Insomnia (Sleeplessness)

A legendary Hollywood comedian once remarked that the only sure way to overcome insomnia is "to get more sleep." Yet sleeplessness is no laughing matter if you're one of the 35 to 50 percent of the population that spends tortured nights twisting and turning, wrestling with the bedding and, then, by dawn's early light, struggling to rise, feeling more tired than when you went to bed.

Recognizing Insomnia

Everyone has nights when, for whatever reason, sleep is hard to come by. Insomnia, however, is considered more of a pattern that may occur over a course of many nights, be it the inability to fall asleep, waking during the night, or some combination of the two.

Women tend to have more trouble with insomnia than men. Single people are more prone to sleeplessness than those who are married. A large percent of divorcees and widowed persons have insomnia. Happy individuals also sleep best, by most accounts.

What Are the Causes of Insomnia?

Reasons for not being able to fall asleep or stay asleep are endless. Here are a few of the most common:

- Uncomfortable bedding
- High noise level
- Too much light in the room
- Pain from illness
- Frequent bathroom trips (caused by an enlarged prostate or bladder infection)
- Anxiety
- Depression
- Stress
- Too much caffeine or other stimulants
- Low blood sugar
- Poor digestion

What You Can Take

For best results, alternate the following sleep aids:

Nutrients

Name	Dosage	Benefits
Calcium	One capsule an hour or two before bedtime	Adequate calcium levels in the blood are required for proper sleep.
Inositol	1,000 mg in the morning and another 1,000 mg an hour before bedtime	Member of the vitamin B-complex family that acts as a sedative.
5-HTP	1,000 mg prior to bedtime	Converts to serotonin, a brain neurotransmitter that produces a calming effect conducive to sleep.
Kava	250 mg before bedtime	Powerful relaxant effects.
Melatonin	1–3 mg daily	Hormone secreted by the pineal gland that has proven highly effective in promoting good sleep.

Herbs

Name	Dosage	Benefits
Chamomile tea	1 cup an hour or two before bedtime	Excellent herb for inducing sleep.
Valerian root	400 mg an hour before bedtime	Induces quicker falling asleep as well as deeper sleep.

What You Can Do

Follow the six rules for beating insomnia and sleeping soundly shared with me by Charles Herrera, eminent sleep authority at Mount Sinai Medical Center in New York City. Pleasant dreams!

✓ Use the bedroom for sleep alone with one exception: love-making. No TV or reading! This focus conditions you to expect and get needed sleep.

✓ Follow a regular day and nighttime schedule of activities to accustom your body and mind to adjust more readily to the sleeping mode at bedtime.

✓ Don't get upset when you can't readily sleep. If you're not asleep in 20 minutes, get out of bed and do something relaxing, like listening to slow and soothing music.

✓ Refrain from drinking caffeine-containing beverages or eating chocolate after 4 P.M. Chocolate contains two stimulants: caffeine and theobromine. Some people are kept wide awake at night even if they have no coffee after the wake-up cup in the morning.

✓ Rise at about the same time every day, even if you're tired—especially if you're a senior citizen.

✓ Avoid taking naps. They can throw off your sleeping-waking rhythms.

And Try This!

Try homeopathic remedies, which are often effective against even the toughest cases of insomnia. Three of the best include arsenicum album, ignatia, and nux vomica.

Did You Know?

A little-considered cause of insomnia is nighttime low blood sugar. The blood sugar level drops at night, a form of stress that activates the adrenal glands and other blood sugar regulatory hormones, an energy stimulant that keeps many would-be sleepers awake. A pre-bedtime snack can often prevent this condition (*see* HYPOGLYCEMIA).

Intermittent Claudication (Poor Circulation in Legs)

Intermittent claudication is a condition in which impaired circulation limits one's ability to walk even a city block without excruciating pain and the need to rest. If left untreated, the pain can become intolerable and gangrene may occur, making amputation necessary.

Recognizing Intermittent Claudication

- Severe pain in legs
- Tingling feeling in legs
- Walking becomes difficult

What Are the Causes of Intermittent Claudication?

- Smoking
- Stress
- Lack of exercise
- Overweight
- Nutritional deficiencies (especially vitamin E)
- Toxic levels of heavy metals in the body

What You Can Take

Nutrients

Name	Dosage	Benefits
Vitamin B-complex	100 mg daily	Necessary for maintaining the biochemical balance of all B vitamins when supplementing with any single B vitamin individually.
Vitamin B$_6$	250 mg daily	Enhances blood circulation.
Vitamin C	500–1,000 mg three times daily	Prevents buildup of harmful plaque in the arteries and promotes healing in already damaged arteries.

Name	Dosage	Benefits
Vitamin E	400–1,200 IU daily	Powerful antioxidant that attacks harmful (LDL) cholesterol and prevents clogged arteries.
Arginine	2 g daily	Increases walking distance.
Chondroitin sulphate	400 mg three times daily	Effectively thins blood, reduces blood fats, and helps maintain smooth and elastic arteries.
Folic acid	5 mg daily	Reduces levels of homocysteine in the blood, a prime risk factor for heart attacks.
Inositol hexaniacinate (a type of niacin)	2 g daily	Increases walking distance.
Lycopene	15 mg twice daily	Super antioxidant that attacks harmful (LDL) cholesterol and prevents clogged arteries.

Herbs

Name	Dosage	Benefits
Garlic (odorless)	1 teaspoon three times daily	Lowers blood pressure and helps prevent abnormal blood clotting.
Ginkgo biloba	40 mg three times daily	Enhances circulation and increases pain-free walking distance.

What You Can Do

✓ Combine supplements with daily exercise (walking is preferable).
✓ Don't smoke.
✓ Work to relieve stress (*see* STRESS).
✓ Maintain healthy body weight (*see* OVERWEIGHT).
✓ Test (hair analysis) for toxic levels of heavy metals such as mercury in the body.

✓ Eat foods high in vitamin C, including rose hips, acerola cherries, guavas, black currants, red peppers, oranges, grapefruit and other citrus fruits, cabbage, papayas, cantaloupe, and tomatoes.

✓ Eat foods high in vitamin E, including sunflower seeds, whole wheat, peanuts, cashews, almonds, walnuts, corn oil, soy oil, soy lecithin, spinach, asparagus, broccoli, oats, and avocados.

And Try This!

Try chelation therapy, a safe and effective means of ridding the body of heavy metals. Chelation therapy can be performed either orally or intravenously and has been used successfully to improve blood circulation. Please consult with a physician trained in this practice, as it requires close medical supervision.

Did You Know?

Chelation treatments—sometimes twenty in all—may correct intermittent claudication in that it removes plaque that blocks blood flow in the legs. Intravenous chelation takes longer, costs more than oral chelation, but proves more effective.

Irritable Bowel Syndrome (Spastic Colon)

Irritable bowel syndrome (IBS) had undermined Bart's promising career and love life. Diarrhea that frequently caused him to dash out of management council meetings contributed to his losing a promotion to vice president of a growing manufacturing firm. Painful colon spasms often doubled him up during candlelight dinners with the woman he wanted to marry. The romance died, and he lived on in pain and alternating and embarrassing diarrhea and constipation. Having endured this illness for almost two years, Bart showed up in my office more than a little depressed—but not for long!

Recognizing Irritable Bowel Syndrome

IBS is a common reason for trips to the doctor. Typical symptoms include:

- Alternating between constipation and diarrhea
- Gas
- Bloating
- Stomach pain
- Nausea
- Vomiting
- Headaches

What Are the Causes of Irritable Bowel Syndrome?

IBS occurs when the muscles controlling the digestive tract fail to contract in unison, either moving waste out too quickly (diarrhea) or too slowly (constipation). Contributing factors may include the following:

- Stress
- Food allergies (especially dairy products and wheat)
- Yeast overgrowth
- Imbalance of friendly and unfriendly bowel organisms
- Overuse of laxatives
- Overuse of antibiotics
- Eating too fast and not chewing food completely
- Viral and bacterial infections
- Poor diet
- Lack of exercise

What You Can Take

Nutrients		
Name	**Dosage**	**Benefits**
Fructo-oligosaccharides (FOS)	2,000 mg daily	Feeds and nurtures friendly bacteria in the colon.
Probiotics (including acidophilus)	Two capsules containing up to 20 billion live cells per unit daily	Feeds and nurtures friendly bacteria in the colon.

Herbs

Name	Dosage	Benefits
Peppermint oil (enteric coated)	Two 0.2 ml capsules between meals	Helpful in managing the symptoms associated with IBS.

What You Can Do

✓ Test for food allergies (*see* ALLERGIES).
✓ Exercise daily (I suggest a 30-minute walk after dinner).
✓ Drink at least 8–10 glasses of pure spring water daily.
✓ Work to relieve stress (*see* STRESS).
✓ Eat plenty of fresh fruits and vegetables.
✓ Eat slowly and chew food completely.
✓ Avoid eating right before bedtime.
✓ Avoid dairy products and wheat.
✓ Avoid sugar and other refined carbohydrates.
✓ Avoid caffeine, alcohol, and carbonated beverages.
✓ Don't smoke.

And Try This!

Closely examine your emotional life. It may prevent irritable bowel syndrome from responding to treatment. A study reported in the Scandinavian journal, Gastroenterology, *reveals that anxiety, depression, and hostility may cause sleeplessness, a condition that worsens irritable bowel syndrome.*

Did You Know?

According to a study published in the prestigious British medical journal *The Lancet*, 66 percent of all patients suffering from irritable bowel syndrome have one or more food allergies.

Kidney Stones

Few conditions spark more fears than kidney stones, especially among those who have had them once and never want to again. Unfortunately, at least half will, as statistics indicate they tend to reoccur in the same people again and again. Kidney stones (also called oxalates) are a combination of calcium and uric acid. They are sharp and vary in size from a grain of sand to a thumbnail. After your kidneys process fluids, they pass them down tubes called ureters that empty into the bladder. Kidney stones can block this flow and create a host of problems, including unimaginable pain!

Recognizing Kidney Stones

Nobody has described the pain of passing kidney stones as well as Patrick Quillin, Ph.D., R.D., in *Healing Nutrients*. He writes that trying to get rid of kidney stones has the "effect of dragging a fish hook through the delicate vessels of the excretory system—very, very painful." Additional symptoms may include:

- Chills
- High fever
- Intense lower back pain
- Nausea

- Abdominal bloating
- Blood in the urine
- Frequent urination

What Are the Causes of Kidney Stones?

Most kidney stones are the result of too much calcium in the blood, which is then absorbed and creates an excess amount of calcium in the urine. It is here that stones are formed. Contributing factors can include the following:

- Family history
- Diet high in sugar and other refined carbohydrates
- Diet high in oxalic acids (mainly from heavy intake of animal proteins)

- Lack of fiber in the diet
- Dehydration
- Urinary tract infections
- Intake of too much vitamin D (excess of 400 IU daily)
- Nutritional deficiencies (especially magnesium)

What You Can Take

Nutrients

Name	Dosage	Benefits
Vitamin A	10,000 IU daily	Helps heal delicate membranes of the urinary tract that can be damaged by kidney stones.
Vitamin B_6	10 mg twice daily	Deficiencies linked to kidney stones. Effective in preventing recurrence of stones when taken with magnesium.
Magnesium	300 mg daily	Reduces absorption of calcium. Effective in preventing recurrence of stones when taken with vitamin B_6.
Zinc	15–30 mg daily	Helps heal delicate membranes of the urinary tract that can be damaged by kidney stones.

What You Can Do

For patients suffering intense pain from kidney stones, I recommend immediate medical treatment, not self-treatment. People have died from this ailment. Ultrasonic shattering of these stones is one of the quickest ways of getting rid of them. However, prevention is the best and most economical method. Here's how:

✓ Drink at least 8–10 glasses of pure spring water daily.
✓ Add more fibrous foods to the diet, including oat bran, pectins, and guar gum.

✓ Avoid oxalic acid foods such as beet tops, chard, chocolate, cocoa, coffee, rhubarb, and spinach.

✓ Avoid sugar and other refined carbohydrates.

✓ Minimize consumption of animal proteins.

✓ Exercise regularly.

✓ Beware of vitamin D intake above 400 IU daily.

✓ Eat foods high in magnesium, including blackstrap molasses, sunflower seeds, wheat germ, almonds, soybeans, Brazil nuts, soy lecithin, pecans, oats, walnuts, whole grains, rice, mushrooms, barley, salmon, corn, avocados, bananas, cheese, and tuna.

✓ Eat foods high in vitamin B_6, including brewer's yeast, brown rice, whole wheat, royal jelly, soybeans, rye, lentils, sunflower seeds, alfalfa, salmon, wheat germ, tuna, bran, walnuts, cashews, peanuts, peas, liver, avocados, beans, turkey, oats, chicken, halibut, lamb, and bananas.

And Try This!

Try drinking diluted lemon juice regularly throughout the day if you are already suffering from stones. It will not only help alleviate the pain, but keep you well hydrated.

Did You Know?

A false and character-assassinating charge was hurled at vitamin C several years ago to the effect that, in large amounts, it may cause kidney stones. This arose from theoretical findings. Worldwide vitamin C authorities found the claim faulty, misleading, and dangerous in discouraging use of vitamin C, which now benefits billions of people. Among those who dissented were Nobel Laureate Linus Pauling and Glen Dettman, one of Australia's foremost researchers in nutrition. Dr. Dettman's objections well represent those of others who cried foul: "Sufficient work has been completed by international scientists to show that the vitamin C–oxalate–kidney stone theory is a myth."

Lead Poisoning

It has been many years since oil companies were told to get the lead out of their gas. And they did. It has been many more years since paint makers were told to get the lead out of their products. They did, too. So this means that you and the rest of us are no longer in danger of lead poisoning. Right? Don't bet your home on it! Lead in the environment has not disappeared. It is still part of the dust on roads, freeways, highways, and city streets or washed into creeks, rivers, lakes, oceans and in rain, drinking water, and crops grown on lead-polluted soil. And it continues to accumulate in our bodies at alarming rates.

Recognizing Lead Poisoning

Everyone is at risk for lead poisoning, but children and pregnant women have been shown to be especially vulnerable. The best way to determine lead levels in the body is to have a hair analysis done that can test for not only lead, but the accumulation of other toxic heavy metals as well. Blood tests are not always as accurate. Symptoms associated with lead poisoning may include:

- Muscle soreness
- Dizziness
- Stomach disorders
- Insomnia
- Arthritis
- Anxiety
- Irritability
- Tremors
- Sudden outbursts or tantrums

- Numbness
- Headaches
- Vision problems
- Blue gums
- Fatigue
- Poor appetite
- Diarrhea
- Learning disabilities
- Metal taste in the mouth

What Are the Causes of Lead Poisoning?

Lead entering the body cannot be distinguished from calcium, and is thus absorbed in the same way, eventually becoming stored in the bones, where it can continue to seep out into other tissues over the course of a lifetime. Since it serves no useful function, the results are never a good thing. Sources of lead in the environment are many. Some of the most widely recognized for their potential to cause problems include the following:

- Leaded gasoline
- Lead-based paints
- Lead pipes (drinking water)
- Imported china, porcelain, and earthenware dishes
- Lead crystal decanters
- Cigarette smoke
- Factory smoke

- Insecticides
- Some cosmetics and hair colorings (check the labels)
- Lead batteries
- Newsprint
- Lead-contaminated soil
- Canned fruit

What You Can Take

Nutrients

Name	Dosage	Benefits
Vitamin B-complex	100 mg daily	Important in preventing nerve damage and neurological disorders caused by lead.
Vitamin C	2,000 mg daily	Helps to remove lead from the body.
Vitamin E	400 IU daily	Antioxidant that protects cells from free radical damage caused by lead.
Calcium	1,000 mg daily	Blocks lead from entering the body. Especially important for pregnant women.
Zinc	30 mg daily	Prevents lead absorption in the body.

What You Can Do

✓ Test (hair analysis) for toxic levels of lead in the body.
✓ Avoid living in pre-1950 homes or apartments with lead-based paint on the walls, or have the paint professionally removed.

✓ Always flush out lead by running the first morning water for 2–3 minutes.

✓ Buy only properly fired glazed china, porcelain, and earthenware dishes.

✓ Never leave wine in crystal decanters for long periods.

✓ Don't smoke.

✓ Eat frequent meals to lower lead absorption.

✓ Avoid a high-fat diet.

✓ Eat foods high in iron, including liver, egg yolk, millet, lentils, walnuts, oats, cashews, whole wheat and rye (never use iron supplements without monitoring from a qualified physician).

✓ Eat foods high in vitamin C, including rose hips, acerola cherries, guavas, black currants, red peppers, oranges, grapefruit and other citrus fruits, cabbage, papayas, cantaloupe, and tomatoes.

✓ Eat foods high in vitamin E, including sunflower seeds, whole wheat, peanuts, cashews, almonds, walnuts, corn oil, soy oil, soy lecithin, spinach, asparagus, broccoli, and avocados.

✓ Eat foods high in calcium, including buttermilk, milk, low fat yogurt, cheddar, parmesan and romano cheeses, carob, brewer's yeast, broccoli, kale, kelp, amaranth, teff, almonds, sesame seeds, and sardines.

✓ Eat foods high in zinc, including seafood, sardines, oysters, soybeans, soy lecithin, kelp, legumes, meat, liver, eggs, brewer's yeast, mushrooms, poultry, whole grains, and pumpkin and sunflower seeds.

✓ Consider chelation therapy, a safe and effective means of ridding the body of toxic heavy metals. Chelation therapy can be performed either orally or intravenously and has been used successfully to treat lead poisoning. Please consult with a physician trained in this practice, as it requires close medical supervision.

And Try This!

Try calling the Culligan Man! The Culligan water company runs a consumer hot line that will direct you to the nearest Culligan dealer for a free testing of your home's water supply for lead (800-285-5442).

Did You Know?

In 1980, environmentalist C. C. Patterson wrote in the *U.S. National Academy of Sciences (NAS) Report* that our total body lead burdens exceed those of our prehistoric ancestors by two to three orders of magnitude, "and typical lead levels in urban air are now up to 10,000 times greater than those found in pre-technological societies." Patterson claimed we are moving irreversibly closer to mass lead poisoning!

Lupus

Lupus is a chronic autoimmune disease (like arthritis), meaning it is a condition in which the body turns on itself and begins to wage war against its own tissue, incorrectly identifying it as a threat. The result is a weakened immune system and a severe state of generalized inflammation that can lead to a host of different problems, including kidney failure and possible heart damage.

Recognizing Lupus

Lupus may strike quickly, within days, or develop slowly over a period of years. The vast majority of cases occur in women under the age of 40 or in children. Symptoms can include:

- Butterfly-shaped red rash over the nose
- Joint pain and inflammation
- Swollen glands
- Fever
- Mouth sores
- Headaches

What Are the Causes of Lupus?

Even lupus authorities are not certain as to the underlying reasons why it occurs. However, they have identified numerous factors that seem either to contribute to its onset or to make the condition worse. These include:

- Stress
- Digestive problems (lack of hydrochloric acid in the stomach)
- Viral or bacterial infections
- Fatigue
- Excessive sun exposure
- Pregnancy
- Vaccination
- Family history
- Food and environmental allergies
- Drug use and reactions to prescription medications
- Toxic levels of heavy metals such as mercury in the body

What You Can Take

Nutrients

Name	Dosage	Benefits
Vitamin C	1,000 mg three times daily	Promotes healing and recharges the immune system.
Vitamin E	600 IU daily	Helps fight against free radicals that damage the immune system and make the condition worse.
Hydrochloric acid	Capsule containing 648 mg of betaine hydrochloride and 130 mg of pepsin	Helpful if there are digestive problems.
Omega-3 fatty acids	1,000 mg three times daily	Protective effects against inflammatory disease.
Zinc	30 mg daily	Strengthens immune systems and promotes healing in general.

Herbs

Name	Dosage	Benefits
Cayenne pepper	20 mg daily	Strengthens immune system and protects integrity of enzyme systems.
Aged garlic	Two 600 mg capsules after each meal	Strengthens immune system and protects integrity of enzyme systems.

Name	Dosage	Benefits
Hawthorn berry	100 mg daily *Warning:* Do not use if you are taking digitalis medications.	Strengthens immune system and protects integrity of enzyme systems.

What You Can Do

✓ Follow a low-fat, low-calorie diet.
✓ Speak to your dentist about replacing mercury fillings with those made of safer materials.
✓ Relieve stress (*see* STRESS).
✓ Test for food and environmental allergies (*see* ALLERGIES).
✓ Test (hair analysis) for toxic levels of heavy metals such as mercury in the body.
✓ Exercise regularly.
✓ Don't smoke.
✓ Avoid processed foods and food additives.
✓ Avoid dairy products.
✓ Avoid alcohol and caffeine.
✓ Avoid vegetables in the nightshade family, including tomatoes, white potatoes, eggplant, and peppers.
✓ Avoid procaineamide, hydraline, anticonvulsants, penicillin, sulfa drugs, and oral contraceptives.
✓ Eat foods high in vitamin C, including rose hips, acerola cherries, guavas, black currants, red peppers, oranges, grapefruit and other citrus fruits, cabbage, papayas, cantaloupe, and tomatoes.
✓ Eat foods high in vitamin E, including sunflower seeds, whole wheat, peanuts, cashews, almonds, walnuts, corn oil, soy oil, soy lecithin, spinach, asparagus, broccoli, oats, and avocados.
✓ Eat foods high in zinc, including seafood, sardines, oysters, soybeans, soy lecithin, kelp, legumes, meat, liver, eggs, brewer's yeast, mushrooms, poultry, whole grains, and pumpkin and sunflower seeds.

And Try This!

*Try eliminating animal fats and omega-6 oils—corn, saf-
flower, and sunflower seed oils—to minimize or prevent
inflammation. Instead take omega-3 fish oils. In a study in
Great Britain, 27 lupus patients on omega-3 fish oils improved. Placebo takers didn't. Andrew Weil, M.D., ad-
vises his lupus patients to eat sardines packed in olive oil
three times a week.*

Did You Know?

A study published in *Clinical Medicine* as far back as 1953
found that 9 out of 12 lupus patients given 100–150 mg capsules of vitamin E after each meal, and receiving 150 mg injections of vitamin E intramuscularly two to three times weekly,
experienced an excellent response.

Lyme Disease

Little brown ticks the size of a pinhead are causing big trouble these days. In grassy or wooded areas throughout the
United States, they're attaching themselves to the skin of
people and spreading Lyme disease. They're most prevalent
in the Northeast and Mid-Atlantic states, the upper Midwest
(Wisconsin and Minnesota), and the West Coast (California
and Oregon).

Recognizing Lyme Disease

What is called a bull's-eye rash—pink to red—centers
around the tick bite within 30 days, accompanied by flu-like
symptoms: chills, fever, headache, muscle and joint pain, and
fatigue. One or more of the following are later consequences:
light sensitivity, facial paralysis, tingling and numbness, stiff

neck, arthritis, swollen knees, memory impairment, dizziness, irregular heartbeat, chest pain, and depression.

What Are the Causes of Lyme Disease?

- Ticks that burrow headlong into human flesh, lodge there, suck blood, and leave harmful spirochete bacteria under the skin

What You Can Take

Nutrients

Name	Dosage	Benefits
Vitamin A	50,000 IU daily for male adults, 10,000 IU max for pregnancy-eligible women, plus 50,000 IU beta-carotene	Boosts immunity.
Vitamin C	500 mg five times daily	Boosts immunity.
Zinc	30 mg daily	Boosts immunity.
Shark liver oil, which contains squalene	570 mg capsules three times a day	Boosts immunity.

Herbs

Name	Dosage	Benefits
Echinacea	200 mg three times daily	Boosts immunity, fights infection.
Astragalus	200 mg three times daily	Boosts immunity.
Garlic (aged, odorless)	400 mg three times daily	Antibiotic action and boosts immunity.

What You Can Do

✓ Avoid heavily wooded and grassy areas, especially in spring and summer.

✓ Wear white garments that make ticks more visible.

✓ Wear a close-fitting hat, a long-sleeved shirt, and long pants, tucked into socks so that ticks can't reach your skin.

✓ After hiking in tick-infested areas, immediately wash clothes in hot water and dry at high heat, and in the nude, check the favorite hiding places of the ticks: armpits, ears, groin, hairline, and behind the knees.

✓ Remove a tick as soon as possible, but always within 24 hours after exposure, the time it takes a tick to transmit sufficient Lyme disease bacteria to cause infection.

✓ Use small tweezers as near as possible to the tick's mouth— the part imbedded in your skin—and gently pull straight backward.

✓ Don't squeeze the tick's body or it will act like a hypodermic needle to inject harmful bacteria into you.

✓ Seal the tick in a container and have your doctor send it to a lab to determine the type of bacteria that it carries.

✓ Eat vitamin C–richest foods—in addition to supplements— guavas, red and green peppers, strawberries, citrus fruits, papayas, elderberries, cantaloupe, loganberries, tomatoes, squash, pineapple, and avocados.

✓ Eat raw garlic frequently for its antibiotic and immune-empowering properties.

✓ Apply a warm/moist compress to the infected area and joints for dull pain.

✓ Apply an ice pack in a plastic bag for 10 minutes at a time for sharp pain. Longer exposure may harm the skin.

✓ Be patient, because symptoms may plague you for weeks or months, even after the infection has cleared up.

And Try This!

Act as soon as you suspect Lyme disease. Delay will prolong the need for treatment. Eat more fresh vegetables and fruits, follow a low-fat diet, and drink fresh produce juices throughout the day. This regimen, along with supplements—vitamins, zinc, and the herbals recommended earlier—has helped my patients overcome Lyme disease quickly.

Did You Know?

The Lyme disease-spreading salivary glands of the poppy seed-size tick are in its belly, so don't be discouraged if you can't remove the insect's mouth from your skin. There is bound to be irritation around any insect bite, because something foreign to your system is still embedded in your skin. This doesn't necessarily indicate that it's Lyme disease unless the irritation is bull's-eye shaped. Studies show that the immune response of some patients is so strong that Lyme disease never develops. However, report to your doctor as soon as possible after a suspicious-looking bite, along with the tick.

Macular Degeneration

In cases of macular degeneration, the macula (a small yellowish part of the retina, the focal point of vision) deteriorates, making objects in the central field of vision blurry, gray, or invisible, while peripheral vision remains. Sometimes colors seem faded. Straight lines of print appear to be wavy and distant highway signs are often illegible.

Macular degeneration is a leading cause of blindness in senior citizens.

Recognizing Macular Degeneration

- Blurred central vision
- Print becomes difficult to read and can appear wavy
- Colors can seem faded

What Are the Causes of Macular Degeneration?

Free radicals, militant molecules that attack the macula, are the cause of macular degeneration. Contributing factors can include:

- Smoking
- Aging
- High blood pressure
- Arteriosclerosis

What You Can Take

Nutrients

Name	Dosage	Benefits
Vitamin A	10,000 IU daily	Required for proper functioning of eyes and good vision.
Vitamin B-complex	100 mg daily	Essential for metabolism of nutrients in the eyes.
Vitamin C	500 mg three times daily	Key antioxidant that fights against free radicals.
Vitamin E	800 IU daily	Potent antioxidant that has shown promising results in macular degeneration patients.
Copper	2 mg daily	Required when taking high doses of zinc.
Lycopene	15 mg twice daily, morning and night	Super antioxidant believed to be 100 times stronger than vitamin E in fighting free radicals.
Ginkgo biloba	40 mg four times daily	Improves blood circulation to the retina.
Selenium	200–300 mcg daily	Most effective when combined with vitamin E.
Taurine	1 g twice daily Note: No protein or amino acids one hour before or after taking.	Most effective when combined with vitamin E.
Zinc picolinate	60 mg daily	Deficiencies have been linked to macular degeneration and other eye conditions.

What You Can Do

✓ Don't smoke.
✓ Avoid alcohol.
✓ Avoid sugar and other refined carbohydrates.
✓ Exercise regularly.
✓ Eat plenty of fresh fruits and vegetables.
✓ Eat foods high in vitamin A, including eggs, milk, cheese, cream, butter, yogurt, salmon, bass, halibut, mackerel, herring, whitefish, sardines, tuna, clams, shrimp, beef, chicken, pistachios, pecans, walnuts, lentils, and soybeans.
✓ Eat foods high in vitamin C, including rose hips, acerola cherries, guavas, black currants, red peppers, oranges, grapefruit and other citrus fruits, cabbage, papayas, cantaloupe, and tomatoes.
✓ Eat foods high in vitamin E, including sunflower seeds, whole wheat, peanuts, cashews, almonds, walnuts, corn oil, soy oil, soy lecithin, spinach, asparagus, broccoli, butter oats, and avocados.
✓ Eat foods high in selenium, including Brazil nuts, fish, organ meats, whole grains, eggs, cabbage, corn, peas, onions, garlic, chicken, beets, barley, and tomatoes.
✓ Eat foods high in zinc, including seafood, sardines, oysters, soybeans, soy lecithin, kelp, legumes, meat, liver, eggs, brewer's yeast, mushrooms, poultry, whole grains, and pumpkin and sunflower seeds.

And Try This!

Taking a daily combination of plant-derived antioxidants—400 mg of bilberry extract and 20 mg of beta carotene—will enlarge your visual field and enhance your night vision. Eating antioxidant-rich fruits and vegetables a minimum of five times weekly can reduce by half the risk of developing macular degeneration.

Did You Know?

In a large-scale study of 31,843 female nurses, results showed that nurses who smoked 25 or more cigarettes a day were 2.4

times more prone to developing macular degeneration than non-smokers. Smoking is notorious for reducing blood circulation.

Memory Loss

Even if your memory retains information like a sieve holds water, there's still hope. Unfortunately, many people—thirty-somethings, the middle-aged, and the elderly—give up too early. They forget a person's name and, in embarrassment, mutter something such as "I must be getting old." Although memory efficiency may decrease as birthdays increase, it's not so much the number of years as the number and degree of abuses endured by the brain during that time. As I have found in my medical practice, low thyroid function, substandard nutrition, and stress lead the list of abuses.

Recognizing Memory Loss

Memory is one of the many activities we take for granted and rarely consider until it isn't there. Forgetting a name or an appointment every now and then is nothing to worry about. It happens to everyone. However, when frustrating patterns begin to develop or you find that you cannot recall things that used to appear with seemingly little effort, you may have cause for concern.

What Are the Causes of Memory Loss?

- Low thyroid function
- Nutritional deficiencies (especially the B vitamins)
- Stress
- Food and environmental allergies (especially dairy products and wheat)
- Toxic levels of heavy metals in the body such as lead and mercury
- Free radical exposure
- Alcohol and drug use
- Yeast overgrowth

What You Can Take

Nutrients

Name	Dosage	Benefits
Vitamin B-complex	100 mg daily	Necessary for maintaining the biochemical balance of all B vitamins when supplementing with any single B vitamin individually.
Vitamin B_3 (niacin)	50–100 mg daily	Has powerful influence on thinking and remembering by dilating arteries and capillaries, making possible efficient blood delivery to the brain.
Vitamin B_{12}	1,000 mcg under the tongue daily	Deficiencies have been linked to a wide array of mental and emotional problems, including memory loss.
Acetyl-L-carnitine	500 mg daily	Increases energy production in brain cells, boosting memory and reversing memory loss in the process.
DMAE	10–20 mg daily	Super brain supplement that increases the production of choline, which is converted into acetylcholine, the memory booster.
Ginkgo biloba	80 mg twice daily	Dilates arteries and capillaries and often brings about a rebirth of memory.
Kelp	500 mg that contains 225 mcg of iodine (the thyroid's favorite food)	Beneficial to first-generation hypothyroids, but not second- or third-generation.
Lecithin	Three capsules daily of 400 mg of low-cost lecithin with 144 mg of phosphatidyl choline	Major ingredient, choline, essential to remembering and learning.

Name	Dosage	Benefits
Phosphatidyl-serine (PS)	300 mg daily	Most remarkable of the newly discovered "brain nutrients." Keeps brain cell membranes soft and flexible, and also increases the number of brain receptor sites, creating additional communication networks.
Pyroglutamic acid	100 mg daily	Helps restore fading memory, especially in alcoholics.
Thyroid hormone	As prescribed by physician	Low thyroid function has been linked to memory loss.

- Low blood sugar
- Chronic fatigue
- Impaired blood flow to the brain
- Serious underlying illness (e.g. Alzheimer's disease, diabetes)

What You Can Do

✓ Relieve stress (*see* STRESS).
✓ Test for low thyroid function (*see* HYPOTHYROIDISM).
✓ Test for food and environmental allergies (*see* ALLERGIES).
✓ Test (hair analysis) for toxic levels of heavy metals in the body.
✓ Exercise regularly.
✓ Don't smoke.
✓ Avoid alcohol, caffeine, and drugs.
✓ Avoid sugar and other refined carbohydrates.
✓ Eat foods high in vitamin B_1, including Brazil nuts, bee pollen, pecans, peas, buckwheat, oats, whole wheat, lentils, brown rice, walnuts, egg yolk, and liver.
✓ Eat foods high in vitamin B_{12}, including liver and other organ meats, fish, cheese, eggs, and legumes.
✓ Add anchovies and sardines to the diet, the only two foods known to contain significant amounts of DMAE.

And Try This!

Try paying attention! Research indicates that simply focusing on something more closely at the time it is happening will help you remember it later.

Did You Know?

Dr. Robert Atkins, writer of many best-selling nutrition books, disclosed results of a double-blind study of 149 volunteers over age 50. Half of the group took 300 mg of phosphatidylserine daily for 3 months. The other half took placebos. Takers of phosphatidylserine averaged a 15 percent improvement in memory and thinking. Individuals with the most impaired memory made the greatest gains. The lead researcher wrote that phosphatidylserine reversed the mental loss by almost 12 years.

Menopause

Some women breeze through menopause as if it weren't there. Others suffer through it with hot flashes, night sweats, drying or irritation of the vagina, osteoporosis, headaches, nervousness, depression, and/or heavy fatigue. Without question, there's a physiological basis for menopausal symptoms. However, additional factors seem to be involved. If they weren't, why do cross-cultural studies reveal that women in many other countries experience few, if any, of these symptoms? It may surprise you to know that hot flashes are virtually unknown in Japan, where there's not even a term for them in the language.

Recognizing Menopause

Menopause, the point at which a woman stops ovulating and menstruating, and is thus no longer fertile, generally begins around age 50. Individual women vary greatly with respect to symptoms associated with menopause. Symptoms, in fact, may not be the right word since menopause is not an illness, but a natural transition period in life. Nevertheless, it is a transition many women wish occurred less dramatically. Common conditions accompanying menopause include the following:

- Hot flashes
- Night sweats
- Drying or irritation of the vagina
- Osteoporosis
- Headaches
- Nervousness
- Depression
- Fatigue
- Dizziness
- Shortness of breath
- Heart palpitations
- Lowered sexual desire

What Are the Causes of Menopause?

The physical changes brought about during menopause are the result of decreased levels of the hormones estrogen and progesterone in the blood. But this may not be the entire story. Some physiologists and psychologists feel that the different perception of menopausal women in our culture—and the deep desire to stay young—help to make physical symptoms of this separation more pronounced.

Other factors known to exacerbate physical symptoms include:

- Low thyroid function
- Low blood sugar
- Stress
- Smoking
- Caffeine
- Alcohol
- Lack of exercise
- Diet high in animal proteins

What You Can Take

Nutrients

Name	Dosage	Benefits
Vitamin E	400-800 IU daily	Offers relief against menopausal symptoms, including hot flashes, night sweats, fatigue, nervousness, heart palpitations, and depression.

Name	Dosage	Benefits
Isoflavones from soybeans	200 mg daily	Natural source of phyto-estrogens that helps to relieve hot flashes, night sweats, and a hardened or infected vagina without the cancer risks associated with taking estrogen.

Herbs

Name	Dosage	Benefits
Black cohosh	40 mg with a strength of 2.5 percent triter-penes taken twice daily with meals	Effective in relieving hot flashes, night sweats, and vaginal dryness.
Chasteberry	225 mg capsule twice daily. (Take with black cohosh for best results.)	Helps relieve hot flashes and sweats.
Sage (garden)	4 tablespoons of the dried product in a hot cup of water	Can prevent night sweats within an hour or two of taking.

Homeopathy

Name	Dosage	Benefits
Cimicifuga racemosa (black cohosh)	6x	Helps deal with hot flashes and night sweats.
Kali carbonicum (potassium carbonate)	6x	Helps to ease depression, irritability, and hypersensitivity associated with menopause.
Onosmodium virgin-anum (false gromwell)	6x	Contributes to restoring sexual vitality, while preventing violent headaches and alleviating fatigue.
Salix nigra (black willow)	6x	Prevents and relieves vaginal dryness.
Sepia (cuttlefish)	6x	Helps deal with hot flashes, vaginal dryness, and menopausal headaches.

What You Can Do

✓ Reject the idea that menopause is an illness, rather than a natural passage into a new phase of life.

✓ Exercise 4 times weekly for about 30 minutes (e.g. hiking, brisk walking, jogging, running, yoga, or dancing).

✓ Drink at least 8–10 glasses of pure spring water daily.

✓ Work to relieve stress (*see* STRESS).

✓ Test for low thyroid function (*see* HYPOTHYROIDISM).

✓ Don't smoke.

✓ Eat plenty of fresh fruits and vegetables, lentils, soybeans, and whole grains.

✓ Eat plenty of foods containing natural phytoestrogens, such as soy, flaxseed, chia seed and oil, nuts, alfalfa, apples, celery, and parsley.

✓ Avoid sugar and other refined carbohydrates.

✓ Avoid caffeine and alcohol.

✓ Minimize consumption of animal proteins.

✓ Apply a mixture of the contents of a 500 mg capsule of evening primrose oil and a 400 IU capsule of vitamin E to prevent or combat vaginal drying.

✓ Apply aloe vera juice to the vagina to cope with infection or irritation and to lubricate it before sex.

And Try This!

Try the natural progesterone cream created by Dr. John R. Lee, a family practitioner in Sebastapol, California. Dr. Lee's cream has been used successfully (and safely) by menopausal women for almost 20 years. It is available in most health food stores.

Did You Know?

A smashing best-seller of more than a generation ago, *Forever Feminine,* by Dr. Robert A. Wilson, tended to isolate menopausal women from the rest of society. Dr. Wilson indicated that menopause is essentially a physical disorder caused by the natural diminishing of estrogen secretion with advancing years and that it is correctable by hormone replacement therapy (HRT). With the bait that estrogen could keep women forever feminine, Dr. Wilson also stated that, due to declining hormones, menopausal women could become "sexless caricatures of their former selves." Thanks to Wilson's persuasive book, menopause came to be regarded as a disease. The medical profession still considers it as such and promotes hormone taking, despite the fact that this can cause a greater frequency of uterus and breast cancer, as well as liver and cardiovascular ailments.

Mercury Toxicity (Fillings and Environmental Exposure)

Everyone who has read *Alice in Wonderland* was introduced to a funny fictional character called the Mad Hatter. Author Lewis Carroll patterned him after real workers who used mercury for shaping felt hats and were anything but funny. They became toxic, dizzy, and acted in such bizarre ways that the expression "mad as a hatter" soon became popular throughout Great Britain. Today, all of us are exposed to mercury, although less evidently and generally not to the degree that the Mad Hatters were. Still, if left unchecked, the accumulation of mercury can be deadly serious, as it's been linked to conditions such as arthritis, multiple sclerosis, Alzheimer's disease, and lupus.

Recognizing Mercury Toxicity

The best way to determine mercury levels in the body is to have a hair analysis test done by a physician. Symptoms of mercury toxicity can include the following:

- Anorexia
- Fatigue
- Dizziness
- Poor coordination
- Numbness
- Memory loss

- Bloody diarrhea
- Depression
- Bad temper
- Dermatitis
- Headaches

- Emotional instability
- Vomiting
- Gum disease
- Loss of hearing
- Loss of vision

What Are the Causes of Mercury Toxicity?

The world's foremost researchers on mercury toxicity agree that the major human exposure to inorganic mercury is from amalgam fillings in teeth. Hundreds of studies by national and international authorities show that mercury vapors come from amalgam fillings while people chew, brush their teeth, eat hot or acidic foods, or grind their teeth nervously (bruxism). Other sources of environmental mercury include:

- Vehicle exhaust
- Talc body powder
- Floor waxes
- Wood preservatives
- Pesticides

- Tattoo inks
- Some oil paints
- Large predator ocean fish such as marlin, sharks, and swordfish
- Shellfish that congregate near shore

What You Can Take

Nutrients

Name	Dosage	Benefits
Vitamin C	500 mg three times daily	An immune system booster that protects against mercury toxicity.
Selenium	200 mcg daily	An antagonist to mercury, neutralizing its effects in the body.

Herbs

Name	Dosage	Benefits
Chorella	Half a capsule to 14 capsules daily	Binds with mercury and helps draw it out of the body.
Garlic (odorless)	600 mg three times daily	Contains compounds that help excrete mercury.

What You Can Do

✓ Avoid all sources of mercury.

✓ Test (hair analysis) for toxic mercury levels in the body.

✓ Speak to your dentist about replacing mercury fillings with those made from safer, nontoxic materials.

✓ Refrain from eating large predator fish (e.g. shark and swordfish) and shellfish that contain mercury.

✓ Drink at least 8–10 glasses of pure spring water daily.

✓ Consume fresh garlic daily.

✓ Eat foods high in vitamin C, including rose hips, acerola cherries, guavas, black currants, red peppers, oranges, grapefruit and other citrus fruits, cabbage, papayas, cantaloupe, and tomatoes.

✓ Eat foods high in selenium, including Brazil nuts, fish, organ meats, whole grains, eggs, cabbage, corn, peas, onions, garlic, chicken, beets, barley, and tomatoes.

✓ Consider chelation therapy, a safe and effective means of ridding the body of toxic heavy metals. Chelation therapy can be performed either orally or intravenously and has been used successfully to treat mercury toxicity. Please consult with a physician trained in this practice, as it requires close medical supervision.

And Try This!

Always broil fish—especially large ocean fish that sometimes contain mercury. Mercury and other toxins are mainly stored in fat, and broiling releases them to the pan below.

Did You Know?

The official position of the American Dental Association is that mercury is so tightly bound in fillings "that only insignificant amounts of it escape." However, in an article in the *Townsend Letter for Doctors,* Dr. Sandra Denton quotes two researchers of poisonous metals at Utah State University—Sharma and Obersteiner: "Mercury is a strong protoplasmic poison that penetrates all living cells of the body . . . the single most toxic metal that we have ever investigated—even in minute concentrations."

Milk Intolerance

A great deal of confusion exists about milk intolerance. Some people think it is an all-or-none condition, that if they suffer from its common symptoms—gas, bloating, or diarrhea—they can't tolerate *any* milk. Some think that they can't eat any dairy products without painful reactions. Still others think that the standard milk tolerance test is always accurate and, if it shows positive results, rules out dairy products for life. These three notions, however, are not *always* true. Problems arise from the fact that most people do not secrete enough of the enzyme lactase to digest milk sugar's lactose—to break it down into glucose and galactose—so that it can be absorbed by the body. Yet there are simple solutions to this problem.

Recognizing Milk Intolerance

The best indicator of milk intolerance is if you regularly experience any of the following symptoms within an hour or two of consuming dairy products other than yogurt:

- Gas
- Diarrhea
- Bloating
- Stomach cramps

What Are the Causes of Milk Intolerance?

Milk intolerance occurs due to a failure to secrete enough lactase, the enzyme responsible for digesting milk sugar. Most adults, in fact, are milk intolerant to some degree, depending on their hereditary background. Usually only those from northern and central European countries, or children or grandchildren of these populations in the United States, Australia, and New Zealand are completely free of the problem.

What You Can Take

Nutrients

Name	Dosage	Benefits
Probiotics (acidophilus)	One capsule containing up to 20 billion live cells daily	Helps colonize intestinal tract with friendly bacteria that promote healthy digestion.
Lactase	One tablet containing 3,000 FFC units and 4 mg of rennin daily	Missing enzyme in milk intolerants that leads to an inability to digest milk sugar.

What You Can Do

✓ Avoid dairy products in general except for yogurt.

✓ If you choose to consume milk or other dairy products, space them over three meals.

✓ Drink milk with lactase added.

✓ Make sure your milk is not from cows given bovine growth hormone and antibiotics.

✓ Eat yogurt freely (not a problem for milk intolerants), but avoid junk food yogurts with sugar and unacceptable additives, or that contain no live acidophilus cultures.

✓ Minimize intake of processed foods (many contain hidden milk ingredients).

✓ Make sure to read labels for hidden milk ingredients in many products—even hot dogs and bologna!

And Try This!

Try using soy milk or rice milk in place of cow's milk. You can also find cheeses made from soy. A good health food store should offer plenty of tasty options, and many large supermarkets now carry soy and rice substitutes for dairy products as well.

Did You Know?

Many people think that milk intolerance is a milk allergy. Actually, they are two different things. Milk intolerance rises from insufficient lactase to digest milk sugar. Milk allergy is an immune system response to allergens in the milk.

Miscarriage

A miscarriage, also referred to as spontaneous abortion, occurs when a pregnancy is not carried to term. Miscarriages are not uncommon, but often are not discussed because of the complex set of emotions that follow from them. Many factors are believed to contribute to miscarriages, but every case has its own unique set of circumstances involved. Obviously, the focus here is on how best to prevent them.

Recognizing Miscarriage

The early warning signs of miscarriage are bleeding and/or cramping during pregnancy. You should contact your doctor immediately in the event of either.

What Are the Causes of Miscarriage?

- Low thyroid function
- Diabetes
- Hormonal imbalance
- Cytomegalovirus
- Chlamydia
- Herpes
- Chromosomal abnormalities
- Anatomical problems of the womb
- Infections
- Fibroids
- Smoking
- Alcohol
- Stress

What You Can Take

Nutrients		
Name	Dosage	Benefits
Vitamin C	500 mg three times daily	Helps to assure capillary integrity, essential to delivery of oxygen, nutrients, and thyroid hormone to body cells of the fetus in the womb.
Vitamin E	400 IU daily	Shown to help prevent miscarriage.

What You Can Do

✓ Test for low thyroid function (*see* HYPOTHYROIDISM).
✓ Work to relieve stress (*see* STRESS).
✓ Don't smoke.
✓ Avoid alcohol and caffeine.
✓ Eat 1 teaspoon of wheat germ oil daily as a natural source of vitamin E.
✓ Eat foods high in vitamin C, including rose hips, acerola cherries, guavas, black currants, red peppers, oranges, grapefruit and other citrus fruits, cabbage, papayas, cantaloupe, and tomatoes.

And Try This!

Try the following anti-miscarriage formula offered by the late herbologist, Dr. John R. Christopher: 1 teaspoon of false unicorn and lobelia in a cup of distilled water to be consumed as a tea throughout the day at the first sign of bleeding during pregnancy.

Did You Know?

There's an old wives' tale that Nature uses spontaneous abortions to reject defective fetuses. A study in the *American Journal of Obstetrics and Gynecology* offers a convincing statistic to the contrary. Out of 12,000 cases of threatened miscarriage, only a slim percentage—1.5%—of the fetuses had serious birth defects. These are highly favorable odds for having a normal and healthy baby.

Mitral Valve Prolapse

Mitral valve prolapse (MVP) is a condition in which the valve in the upper left chamber of the heart is deformed or weak and doesn't close properly. There's a leakage that sounds like a heart murmur on the doctor's stethoscope.

Recognizing Mitral Valve Prolapse

An unusual aspect of MVP is that most patients with this condition have no symptoms. However, subtle symptoms for a small minority of such patients include the following:

- Fatigue
- Dull chest pain
- Headache
- Irregular heartbeats
- Slight nervousness
- Low blood pressure
- Slight dizziness

What Are the Causes of Mitral Valve Prolapse?

Authorities on the subject fail to mention a cause of MVP, only that women are three times more likely than men to develop this condition and that people with certain physical characteristics seem the most likely candidates for MVP: those with a depressed breastbone, with curvature of the spine, an unusually straight spine, greater than normal joint flexibility, and being thin and lightweight.

What You Can Take

Nutrients

Name	Dosage	Benefits
Coenzyme Q-10	60 mg three to four times daily	Improves symptoms and strengthens daily heart action.
Magnesium	400 mg three times daily	Helps generate energy for the heart and regularize its beat.

Herbs

Name	Dosage	Benefits
Garlic (aged)	400 mg three times daily	Acts as an antibiotic when the mitral valve is infected.

What You Can Do

✓ Avoid caffeine.
✓ Reduce or eliminate sugar intake.
✓ Avoid hypoglycemia attack with snack in midafternoon.
✓ Abstain from dieting.
✓ Drink 8–9 glasses of spring water daily.
✓ Take part in regular aerobic exercises: bicycling, jogging, swimming, walking.

And Try This!

Be calm in dealing with MVP. The majority of patients live long lives, despite this condition. However, many doctors report that fear and a negative attitude have started panic attacks that make symptoms more intense than they have to be.

Did You Know?

In a study by P. H. Langsjoen, M.D., known for his trailblazing research in cardiomyopathy, volunteers with MVP took 60 mg of coenzyme Q-10 three to four times daily. Results showed that their symptoms improved, and they experienced a bonus value. The abnormal thickness of their heart wall decreased. An increase in thickness tells the cardiologist the heart is working harder than it should.

Motion Sickness and Morning Sickness

What do an afternoon at sea and being pregnant have in common? Well, often an upset stomach, queasiness, nausea, and vomiting, to name just a few things. Motion sickness and morning sickness share the same symptoms, can be set off by similar conditions, and they respond to similar treatments. That's why I've grouped them together here.

Recognizing Motion Sickness and Morning Sickness

- Upset stomach
- Queasiness
- Nausea
- Vomiting
- Headaches
- Dizziness
- Weakness

What Are the Causes of Motion Sickness and Morning Sickness?

- Diet high in saturated fats (both)
- Anxiety (both)
- Nutritional deficiencies (both)
- Empty stomach (both)
- Movement that interferes with the sense of balance maintained by brain and inner ear (motion sickness)
- Eating before traveling (motion sickness)
- Alcohol (motion sickness)

What You Can Take

Nutrients

Name	Dosage	Benefits
Vitamin B_6	10–25 mg three times daily	Studies show it can improve nausea and dizziness resulting from both pregnancy and from a difficulty in keeping one's balance.

Herbs

Name	Dosage	Benefits
Ginger root	Capsule containing half a teaspoon daily	Highly effective remedy for nausea, vomiting, and dizziness that has been used the world over for centuries.

What You Can Do

✓ Avoid a diet high in saturated fats.
✓ Avoid alcohol (especially when pregnant).
✓ Eat mild, lighter foods when traveling or during bouts of morning sickness.
✓ Snack on cheese and crackers in the morning or when traveling.

And Try This!

Try traveling at night if you suffer from motion sickness. It helps reduce the amount of visual stimuli that can result in mixed signals being sent to the brain and the organs of balance in the inner ear.

Did You Know?

An interesting contest was held some years ago by Brigham Young University researchers to find out whether the popular drug Dramamine or the folk remedy ginger root would be more effective in coping with motion sickness. In this double-blind study, student volunteers prone to motion sickness were placed into three groups: (1) those given a capsule containing half a teaspoon of ginger root supplement; (2) those given Dramamine; and (3) those given a look-alike placebo. Strapped into tilting chairs and blindfolded, the students were spun around for as many revolutions as they could endure within a time limit of 6 minutes. Ginger root powder scored a smashing victory! More than half of the volunteers on ginger root lasted for the full 6 minutes. Not a single Dramamine taker was able to last that long.

Night Blindness

There's no mystery as to what night blindness is. It is not being able to see well in the dark of night—or at all—after leaving a building that's brightly lighted. Night blindness should not be accepted casually, because it sometimes leads to an even more critical eye defect: retinitis pigmentosa, a slow deterioration of the retina that can lead to a total loss of sight. Not surprisingly, night blindness is a leading cause of highway accidents.

Recognizing Night Blindness

Difficulty seeing at night is the obvious sign of night blindness. A visit to the optometrist is the only way to know if you are suffering from the condition for sure.

What Are the Causes of Night Blindness?

- Vitamin A deficiency
- Zinc deficiency
- Lack of protein in the diet
- Stress
- Alcohol
- Low thyroid function

What You Can Take

Nutrients

Name	Dosage	Benefits
Vitamin A	10,000 IU daily	Deficiencies are the primary cause of night blindness.
Zinc	30 mg daily	Enables vitamin A to deal with this condition.

Herbs

Name	Dosage	Benefits
Bilberry extract	40-60 mg twice daily	Enhances night vision.

What You Can Do

✓ See an optometrist at the first signs of impaired night vision.
✓ Test for low thyroid function (*see* HYPOTHYROIDISM).
✓ Relieve stress (*see* STRESS).
✓ Avoid alcohol.
✓ Eat protein in eggs, cheese, meat, fish, and poultry.
✓ Eat foods high in vitamin A, including eggs, milk, cheese, cream, butter, yogurt, salmon, bass, halibut, mackerel, herring, whitefish, sardines, tuna, clams, shrimp, beef, chicken, pistachios, pecans, walnuts, lentils, and soybeans.
✓ Eat foods rich in zinc, including herring, wheat germ, blackstrap molasses, liver, sunflower seeds, egg yolk, lamb, chicken, brewer's yeast, oats, and whole wheat.

And Try This!

Make sure to take your vitamin A in foods and/or supplements and zinc at the same time—morning, noon or night, because they work together. Research has established that the enzyme that changes vitamin A to its active form can't work its magic without zinc.

Did You Know?

A fortunate discovery helped make the world aware that the bilberry, a relative of the blueberry, helps make night vision more acute. During World War II, pilots in Britain's Royal Air Force found that their vision was more keen on nights after they ate bilberry jam on their bread. So they made it a regular part of their night missions. In recent years, research indicates that bilberry may be helpful in preventing other eye disorders—cataracts, macular degeneration, and possibly even glaucoma.

Nosebleeds

You've had one, probably more than one, and odds are you've tried to stop it in exactly the wrong way, by leaning your head back and stuffing cotton up your nose. Nosebleeds can happen for all kinds of reasons and they are rarely serious. Still, bleeding of any kind is bad news and needs to be handled quickly and effectively.

Recognizing Nosebleeds

A nosebleed will never go unnoticed!

What Are the Causes of Nosebleeds?

A punch in the nose pretty well tells a person the cause of his nosebleed. Numerous other causes may not be so easy to determine. Common examples include the following:

- Injury
- Colds and nasal swelling
- Blowing the nose too hard
- Picking
- Capillary fragility in the nostrils
- Drying out of nasal membranes in a desert climate
- High blood pressure
- Hemophilia
- Infections
- Overuse of antibiotics or aspirin
- Changes in atmospheric pressure
- Alcohol

What You Can Take

Nutrients

Name	Dosage	Benefits
Vitamin C	1,000 mg and 500 mg of flavonoids three times daily	Prevents nosebleeds by strengthening capillaries, making them less fragile and susceptible to rupture.
Probiotics (including	One capsule containing up to 20 billion live	Helps colonize intestinal tract with friendly bacteria that

| acidophilus) | cells twice daily | promote healthy digestion and absorption of nutrients. |
| Chlorophyll | 1 tablespoon daily or a 100 mcg of vitamin K tablet for a month | Good source of vitamin K, which stops bleeding by inducing normal clotting. |

Homeopathy

Name	Dosage	Benefits
Arnica	30c every fifteen minutes	Stops bleeding.
Belladonna	30c every fifteen minutes	Especially useful for stopping sudden and profuse bleeding.
Hamamelis	30c every fifteen minutes	Stops the flow of profuse but slow bleeding.

What You Can Do

✓ Two of the most common things people do to treat a nosebleed are of no help: (1) putting pressure on the bridge of the nose and (2) holding the head back. Pressure should be applied to the front of the nose because almost all bleeds occur in the fore part. Holding the head back merely keeps the blood from coming out the nose. It drains down the throat. To stop bleeding, it is best to blow the nose gently to remove clots, then to apply pressure to the front part of the nasal passage for 5 to 10 minutes, while breathing through the mouth. Bending a small ice bag around and over the forepart of the nose usually helps as well.

✓ Eat plenty of fresh fruits and vegetables, including citrus fruit and buckwheat, from which the bioflavonoid rutin is derived. Other good dietary sources of bioflavonoids include onions, grains, nuts, soy, and green tea.

✓ Eat a pint of yogurt daily containing live lactobacillus acidophilus.

✓ Limit use of antibiotics and aspirin.

✓ Avoid alcohol.

✓ Always see a doctor immediately for heavy bleeding from any source.

And Try This!

Try to avoid blowing your nose for as long as possible once the bleeding stops. Blowing your nose may just blow out the clots that stopped the bleeding to begin with, leaving you right back where you started.

Did You Know?

Nosebleeds are often more frequent in the winter due to indoor heating. Such conditions make for unusually dry air, an irritant to the inside of the nose that can induce bleeding.

Osteomalacia (Bone Softening)

Osteomalacia is a condition characterized by a softening of the bones brought about by a deficiency in vitamin D. It is also referred to as rickets when occurring in children. While related, osteomalacia is not the same as osteoporosis, the latter being a severer weakening and deteriorating of the bones. Osteomalacia is reversible through dietary interventions, but can lead to serious problems if left untreated, including bending ribs, bowlegs, knock-knees, and scoliosis.

Recognizing Osteomalacia

Osteomalacia is most common among women (especially while pregnant) and children. Early symptoms may include:

- Leg cramps
- Irritability
- Heavy sweating
- Numbness of hands and feet
- Tooth decay

What Are the Causes of Osteomalacia?

A deficiency of vitamin D is the cause of osteomalacia. Contributing factors can include:

- Low dietary intake
- Poor digestion leading to inadequate vitamin D absorption
- Not enough exposure to sunlight

What You Can Take

Nutrients

Name	Dosage	Benefits
Vitamin A	10,000 IU daily	Contributes to the forming and maintenance of strong bones.
Vitamin C	500 mg three times daily	Contributes to the forming and maintenance of strong bones.
Vitamin D	800 IU daily for two weeks for the very deficient and then 400 IU daily	Deficiencies are the cause of osteomalacia.
Calcium	1,000 mg daily	Helps remineralize softened bones.
Magnesium	500 mg daily	Contributes to the forming and maintenance of strong bones.

What You Can Do

✓ Eat foods high in vitamin D, including sardines, salmon, tuna, eggs, mushrooms, sunflower seeds, liver, butter, and cheese.
✓ Consume a tablespoon of cod liver oil twice a week (high in vitamin D).
✓ Drink at least 2 glasses of nonfat milk daily if not milk intolerant or allergic.
✓ Be aware that cathartics, mineral oil, anticonvulsants, and the cholesterol-lowering drug cholestyramine can cause a deficiency of vitamin D.

✓ Increase exposure to natural sunlight to at least 15–20 minutes per day.
✓ Avoid sugar and other refined carbohydrates.

And Try This!

Try this for enhanced calcium absorption if you're having bone problems and suspect your stomach isn't secreting enough hydrochloric acid. Under such circumstances, you may be absorbing only about 4 percent of the calcium carbonate you ingest. Why not buy soluble and ionized calcium citrate, calcium gluconate, or calcium lactate? Then, even with little stomach acid, you'll absorb as much as 45 percent of it.

Did You Know?

A little more than 100 years ago, London was noted for people with many bone disorders. Quite far north, London, with its pall of coal smoke, row upon row of tall buildings, and narrow streets where sunlight could hardly enter, was an ideal city for conditions such as osteomalacia.

Osteoporosis

Estimates are that more than 20 million Americans suffer to some degree from osteoporosis. And most of these are older women. Even worse than these alarming numbers is the fact that many who take calcium supplements to prevent or reverse osteoporosis, weak and honeycombed bones, are unknowingly sabotaging themselves. You could be one of them. If so, you're not to blame, because articles and books on osteoporosis rarely tell you that all calcium products are not created equal. Let's correct these sins of omission.

Recognizing Osteoporosis

Osteoporosis usually takes place in a specific order, according to the research of Cornell University's Lennart Krook and Leo Litvak. It starts with loss of calcium in the jawbone with shrinkage there and in supporting bone drawing away from the teeth (loosening and irritating them, often to the point of bleeding). Next it affects the ribs and vertebrae, and, finally, arm and leg bones. Adding insult to injury is the problem that there are rarely any other noticeable symptoms of such bone loss until the damage has been done. It is often the case that osteoporosis is detected only after a bone is broken due to a fall or some other type of accident.

What Are the Causes of Osteoporosis?

- Inadequate intake and/or absorption of calcium
- Marginal to poor nutrition
- Poor digestion
- Lack of exercise
- Not enough exposure to sunlight
- Lack of the female hormones estrogen and progesterone (postmenopausal women)

- Diet too high in animal proteins and sugar
- Alcohol
- Caffeine
- Overuse of antacids
- Smoking
- Family history

What You Can Take

Nutrients

Name	Dosage	Benefits
Vitamin A	10,000 IU daily	Required for the tearing down of old bone cells and the forming of new ones.
Vitamin B-complex	100 mg daily	Necessary for maintaining the biochemical balance of all B vitamins when supplementing with any single B vitamin.

Name	Dosage	Benefits
Vitamin B$_6$	50 mg daily	Adds strength to connective tissue that supports the bones.
Vitamin B$_{12}$	1,000 mcg under the tongue daily	Promotes normal bone growth.
Vitamin C	500 mg three times daily	Transports calcium to where it is most needed by bones.
Vitamin D	400 IU daily	Essential to the absorption of calcium. Deficiencies directly linked to osteoporosis.
Vitamin K	100 mcg daily	Attracts calcium. Essential to bones being formed, repaired, and rebuilt.
Boron	4 mg daily	Enhances calcium absorption.
Calcium	1,200–1,500 mg daily for those 11 to 24 years old; 1,000 mg daily for women 25 to 50; 1,000–1,500 mg daily for postmenopausal women; and 800 mg daily for adult men	Deficiencies directly linked to osteoporosis.
Copper	3 mg daily	Promotes absorption of minerals critical to healthy bones.
Folic acid	400 mcg daily	Helps to transform hazardous homocysteine (which causes osteoporosis and heart disease) into a harmless substance.
Magnesium	400 mg daily	Helps retain calcium, change vitamin D into its active form, and activate enzyme essential to creating new calcium crystals in bones.
Manganese	5–10 mg daily	Helps to metabolize other key bone minerals, and synthe-

| Manganese (cont'd) | | size connective tissue in bone and cartilage. |
| Zinc | 15–30 mg daily | Enhances calcium absorption. |

What You Can Do

✓ Eat foods high in bioavailable calcium, including kale, kelp, broccoli, brewer's yeast, buttermilk, milk, low fat yogurt, cheddar, parmesan and romano cheeses, carob, amaranth, teff, almonds, sesame seeds, and sardines.

✓ Note that although dairy products may be high in calcium, they are not necessarily the best dietary sources since their calcium is not easily absorbed by the body.

✓ Avoid the use of antacids. They contain aluminum and impair calcium absorption.

✓ Take calcium supplements just before bedtime after a glass of milk or other calcium-rich food (absorbed the best at night).

✓ Perform weight-bearing exercises daily for better bone absorption of calcium.

✓ Increase exposure to natural sunlight to at least 15–20 minutes per day.

✓ Don't smoke.

✓ Avoid alcohol, caffeine, and soft drinks.

✓ Avoid sugar and other refined carbohydrates.

✓ Limit intake of animal proteins.

✓ Eat foods high in vitamin C, including rose hips, acerola cherries, guavas, black currants, red peppers, oranges, grapefruit and other citrus fruits, cabbage, papayas, cantaloupe, and tomatoes.

✓ Eat foods high in vitamin D, including cod liver oil, eggs, herring, organ meats, salmon, and sardines.

And Try This!

Take most of your calcium before bedtime. That's when you'll absorb it best, says Morris Notelovitz, M.D., a calcium researcher. At that time, calcium doesn't have to compete with other nutrients. Also, levels of blood calcium are lowest, so the rate of calcium absorption is highest.

Did You Know?

A study at the Chelsea Soldier's home near Boston demonstrated the importance of vitamin D. Elderly guests showed a marked lack of calcium when they were required to stay indoors for seven consecutive weeks. Their ability to assimilate calcium plunged by 60 percent! Not a good statistic for anyone trying to prevent osteoporosis.

Overweight

For the first time in U.S. history, overweight people outnumber those of normal weight. That's straight from a government scorekeeper, Katherine Flegal, of the National Center for Health Statistics. Things get personal when the bathroom scale, the full-length mirror, and a closet full of tight clothes tell you that you're among the majority. They get frightening, too, because overweight can invite every physical ailment from A to Z, including major ones such as diabetes, high blood pressure, and heart attacks.

Recognizing Overweight

Knowing when those few extra pounds are more than just a few is hardly an exact science. Historically, overweight (or obesity) has been determined by comparing an individual against national weight averages for others of similar age, height, sex, and build. However, a more meaningful measure is to determine your own percentage of body fat. Many health clubs now have equipment to do precisely this. Otherwise, a weight loss center or physician can usually measure it for you. In general, anything below 25 percent is considered healthy in women. In men, the figure is anything below 17 percent.

What Are the Causes of Overweight?

Weight control expert Dr. Albert J. Stunkard, of the University of Pennsylvania, sums it up best: "It's just eating too much. Physical activity hasn't increased enough to make up for it." Sound simple? Well, in most cases it is! But there may be other contributing factors. Some of the most common include:

- Low thyroid function
- Lack of exercise
- Diabetes
- Low blood sugar
- Food allergies (especially dairy products and wheat)

- Nutritional deficiencies
- Stress
- Depression
- Family history
- Crash diets

What You Can Take

Nutrients

Name	Dosage	Benefits
Conjugated linoleic acid (CLA)	Two 300 mg liquid gel units before each meal	Prevents unwanted weight gain, promotes loss of body fat, and increases lean muscle mass.
GTF chromium	One 250 mcg tablet daily *Warning:* Diabetics should take chromium only under the supervision of a physician.	Stabilizes blood sugar, decreasing the craving for sweets. Promotes lean muscle mass and reduces body fat.
Hydroxymethyl Butyrate (HMB)	3 g daily	Promotes weight loss and increases lean muscle mass.
5-HTP	100 mg taken before every meal	Reduces the desire for food.
Hydrocitric acid (HCA)	500 mg taken three times daily	Suppresses appetite and promotes weight loss.
Kelp	One tablet containing 225 mcg of iodine	Speeds up metabolism.
L-carnitine	One 500 mg capsule daily	Boosts energy and endurance, resulting in increased physical activity.

Name	Dosage	Benefits
Pyruvate	3–4 g daily	Speeds up resting metabolic rate.
Thyroid hormone	As prescribed by physician	Speeds up metabolism.

What You Can Do

✓ Exercise strenuously for 30 minutes or more daily with your doctor's permission. Recruit a partner if you find it tough to stick with the program. The Buddy System works best!

✓ Drink at least 8–10 glasses of pure spring water daily.

✓ Eat as many fresh foods as possible—especially fruits, vegetables, and whole grains.

✓ Eat nutrition-dense foods like meat, fish, and eggs, while cutting down on fats.

✓ Eat six or seven small meals daily with the same total calorie count as your usual three meals.

✓ Avoid skipping meals, especially breakfast.

✓ Avoid sugar and other refined carbohydrates.

✓ Avoid processed foods.

✓ Avoid alcohol.

✓ Increase fiber intake up to 30–40 grams daily. The best sources include guar gum, wheat bran and oat bran.

✓ Test for low thyroid function (*see* HYPOTHYROIDISM).

✓ Test for food allergies (*see* ALLERGIES).

And Try This!

Try eating a hearty breakfast very early in the morning; a moderate, late morning lunch; and a light dinner not later than 3:00 P.M. Even if you can't stick to the schedule exactly, the key rule is to allow an 8-hour interval between your last meal (including snacks) and going to bed. You might just be amazed by the results!

Did You Know?

The average American diet includes way too much fat—approximately 38 to 40 percent—so reducing fat by just 10 percent can slash caloric intake. Fat contains 9 calories per gram, in contrast with protein and carbohydrates, which contain just 4 calories per gram.

Pellagra

It's strange that pellagra, a disease identified about 250 years ago, and with a known cure for more than 75 years, is still with us. There are two main reasons for this. Most doctors believe it has been wiped out, so they fail to diagnose and treat it. Second, pellagra now manifests itself only in a nonfatal, subclinical form with symptoms common to many other present-day medical disorders. Its name comes from the Italian "pelle agra," meaning rough skin. However, rough skin is just part of classic pellagra.

Recognizing Pellagra

Classical pellagra was summarized by the four D's: dermatitis, diarrhea, dementia, and death. Symptoms recognized by the medical community today remain consistent with these four D's:

- Red or brownish-red skin (similar to sunburn)
- Skin then becomes rough and scaly
- Headaches
- Inflamed and swollen tongue
- Intestinal pain and distress
- Diarrhea
- Partial paralysis of legs or arms
- Irritability
- Forgetfulness
- Inability to think clearly
- Psychotic behavior similar to schizophrenia

What Are the Causes of Pellagra?

Pellagra is caused by deficiencies in vitamin B_3 (niacin), vitamin B_6, and the amino acid tryptophan. Factors contributing to such deficiencies include the following:

- Vegetarian diet
- Diet highly dependent on corn
- Diet high in processed foods
- Diet high in sugar and other refined carbohydrates (especially white flour)
- Poverty

What You Can Take

Nutrients

Name	Dosage	Benefits
Vitamin B-complex	100 mg daily	Deficiencies in vitamin B$_3$ and vitamin B$_6$ are directly linked to pellagra.

What You Can Do

✓ Avoid processed foods.
✓ Avoid sugar and other refined carbohydrates.
✓ Eat foods high in B vitamins, including fresh fruits and vegetables, beans, nuts and seeds, and whole grain cereals.
✓ Eat foods high in protein such as eggs, meat, and milk.
✓ Eat foods high in tryptophan, including turkey, chicken, milk, salmon, brown rice, lentils, peanuts, pumpkin, and sesame seeds.

And Try This!

If 100 mg of vitamin B-complex causes you to develop flushed, warm, itchy skin due to the amount of niacin in the formula, and you don't want to put up with 15 to 20 minutes of such discomfort, try a 50 mg formula. If that doesn't help, try a 25 mg B-complex. Some companies are still making B-complex in this amount.

Did You Know?

For many years, early in the twentieth century, Dr. Joseph Goldberger, of the U.S. Public Health Service, studied pellagra among the poor in the rural southeastern United States. He concluded that this was a deficiency disease of people whose main food was corn. A diet of eggs, meat, milk, and fresh produce always reversed the condition. He fought an uphill battle to convince others of his findings. After Goldberger's death in 1928, subsequent researchers discovered the specific dietary deficiencies that brought on pellagra.

Premenstrual Syndrome (PMS)

When Eve did what she shouldn't have done in the Garden of Eden, she was told that her sorrow would be multiplied. One of those sorrows had to be premenstrual syndrome (PMS)—a collection of symptoms afflicting women usually beginning a week or two prior to the start of menstruation. If you suffer from PMS, you could berate Eve from here to eternity, but this wouldn't help. So let's look at positive ways of dealing with PMS.

Recognizing PMS

As most graduates from puberty know, there is a long list (too long) of PMS symptoms. Some of the most common include the following:

- Abdominal cramps
- Anxiety
- Bloating
- Breast tenderness
- Confusion
- Crying spells
- Depression

- Dizzziness
- Water retention
- Headache
- Irritability
- Food cravings
- Mood swings

What Are the Causes of PMS?

- Nutritional deficiencies
- Family history
- Stress

- Hormonal imbalances
- Diet high in animal fats
- Diet high in sugar and other

- Alcohol
- Caffeine
- Lack of exercise

Refined carbohydrates
- Low blood sugar

What You Can Take

Nutrients

Name	Dosage	Benefits
Vitamin B-complex	100 mg daily	Vitamin B$_6$ increases absorption of magnesium and discourages water retention.
Vitamin E	400 IU daily	Eases cramps and can reduce breast swelling.
Calcium	300 mg daily	Reduces severity of PMS symptoms.
Evening primrose oil	500 mg three times daily	Highly effective in both relieving and preventing symptoms associated with PMS.
Magnesium	300 mg daily	Relaxes nervous tension and relieves cramps associated with PMS.
Manganese	3–5 mg daily	Reduces severity of PMS symptoms.

What You Can Do

✓ Exercise daily (I suggest a 30-minute walk).
✓ Relieve stress (*see* STRESS).
✓ Drink at least 8–10 glasses of pure spring water daily.
✓ Don't smoke.
✓ Avoid crash diets.
✓ Avoid sugar and other refined carbohydrates (especially white flour).
✓ Avoid salt.
✓ Avoid alcohol, caffeine, and carbonated drinks.
✓ Eat 2 ounces of protein daily (white turkey meat or red meat) and include many complex carbohydrates and fibrous foods over six small meals throughout the day.

✓ Eat at least 1 pint of unsweetened yogurt daily with a teaspoon of brewer's yeast mixed in.
✓ Eat foods high in potassium, including almonds, avocados, bananas, cabbage, cantaloupe, legumes, lentils, parsley, peas, pecans, potatoes, sesame seeds, and sunflower seeds.
✓ Eat foods high in calcium, including buttermilk, yogurt (low fat), cheddar, parmesan and romano cheeses, carob, brewer's yeast, kale, kelp, broccoli, amaranth, teff, almonds, sesame seeds, and sardines.

And Try This!

Try angelica, the most popular women's herb in Asia for PMS, which is especially helpful if you suffer painful menstruation. Best results, under these conditions, come when you start taking it on Day 14 until the end of the menstrual period. It comes in three forms—powdered root, tincture, or fluid extract. The powdered root—1–2 g three times daily—can be mixed in water or milk or made into a tea. The tincture calls for a teaspoon three times a day and the fluid extract (highly concentrated) 1/4 teaspoon, also three times daily.

Did You Know?

Dr. M. G. Brush, of St. Thomas Hospital in London, perhaps the world's largest PMS clinic, administered two 500 mg capsules of evening primrose oil three times a day to 70 women who derived no relief from other forms of treatment. Sixty-seven percent of these patients attained full relief from PMS symptoms and 22 percent gained partial relief. That's a total of 89 percent who benefited—a stunning result!

Prostate Enlargement

It surprises me that so many effective natural treatments for prostate enlargement are so little known. The prostate gland itself surrounds the urethra, the neck of the bladder. It supplies a milky white fluid that contains sperm and is ejaculated at sexual climax. Most men don't give their prostate gland a thought until it starts enlarging, a serious condition called benign prostatic hyperplasia (BPH).

Recognizing Prostate Enlargement

Nearly half of all men over the age of 50 experience prostate enlargement to some degree. Typical symptoms include:

- Difficulty in starting to urinate
- Burning or pain during urination
- A narrower stream
- Possible dribbling, instead of flowing
- More frequent urges to urinate
- Bladder infection
- An unpleasant feeling that the bladder hasn't been completely emptied (it hasn't)

A later stage can bring pain and frustration: the prostate tightening like a vise, further reducing or cutting off the ability to urinate while the powerful need is there. The patient often ends up in a hospital emergency room, where a catheter is inserted, pressing back the prostate and bringing relief. Symptoms of BPH are also similar to those of prostate cancer, and so contact a urologist at the first sign of trouble.

What Are the Causes of Prostate Enlargement?

- Hormonal changes associated with aging
- Nutritional deficiencies (especially zinc)
- High cholesterol

What You Can Take

Nutrients

Name	Dosage	Benefits
Vitamin E	800 IU daily	Reduces prostate enlargement.
Beta sitosterol	20 mg three times daily	Reduces prostate enlargement and improves urine flow.
Lycopene	15 mg twice daily	Super antioxidant that promotes prostate health and protects against prostate cancer.
Omega-3 fatty acids	One 500 mg softgel daily	Reduces prostate enlargement.
Zinc	30 mg daily	Reduces prostate enlargement.

Herbs

Name	Dosage	Benefits
Pygeum Africanum	100 mg capsule daily	Reduces prostate enlargement and increases urine flow.
Saw palmetto	160 mg capsule two to three times daily	Most effective supplement to be used for reducing prostate enlargement and promoting overall prostate health.
Urtica dioica (nettle)	120 mg capsule twice daily	Increases the volume and maximum flow of urine.
Swedish flower pollen extract	Four 250 mg tablets twice daily	Promotes healthy prostate function.

What You Can Do

- ✓ Have a prostate exam once every year.
- ✓ Report even slight bleeding to your doctor.
- ✓ Avoid alcohol and caffeine.
- ✓ Don't smoke.
- ✓ Exercise regularly.

✓ Eat foods high in lycopene, including tomatoes, watermelon, and red grapefruit.
✓ Eat foods high in vitamin E, including sunflower seeds, whole wheat, peanuts, cashews, almonds, walnuts, corn oil, soy oil, soy lecithin, spinach, asparagus, broccoli, oats, and avocados.
✓ Eat foods high in zinc, including seafood, sardines, oysters, soybeans, soy lecithin, kelp, legumes, meat, liver, eggs, brewer's yeast, mushrooms, poultry, whole grains, and pumpkin and sunflower seeds.

And Try This!

Try eating one or two handfuls of sunflower seeds and pumpkin seeds per day. They are high in essential fatty acids, which studies have shown contribute to a reduction in prostate size.

Did You Know?

An enlarged prostate can lead to prostate cancer. A wonderful new herbal formula called PC SPES, consisting of eight herbs, is extremely effective in treating prostate cancer, as well as dramatically reducing PSA scores. (PSA scores are a valuable indicator of prostate cancer activity.) Additional supplements for prostate cancer are: lycopene, selenium, CoQ-10, shark liver oil, flax oil, an herbal astragalus extract in a special form (see resource section), and a food state multi-vitamin mineral.

Pruritus Ani (Anal Itching)

Some years ago an ad for a patent medicine appeared in the back pages of many newspapers. Its headline asked the pertinent and personal question, "Tormented by Rectal Itch?" Although millions are troubled and embarrassed by pruritus ani—a socially acceptable name—I have yet to see a book dealing with natural healing cover this disorder, possibly because nobody dies from it. So here it is.

Recognizing Pruritus Ani

The disorder brings mild and tolerable itching at first. Then it grows in intensity, because the skin is super tender due to many sensitive nerves there. Scratching through clothing causes underwear to "sandpaper" the delicate skin, compounding the problem. Itching can turn to burning and more scratching.

What Are the Causes of Pruritus Ani?

Anal itching occurs when this particular area of tender skin becomes irritated. Factors that can contribute to such irritation include the following:

- Frequent elimination of waste
- Toilet paper that isn't soft enough
- Suppositories
- Enemas
- Soap and water
- Friction from underwear
- Colonization of bacteria and yeast
- High intake of citrus fruits and juices

What You Can Take

Nutrients

Name	Dosage	Benefits
Vitamin A	10,000 IU daily	Contributes to healing of delicate skin and mucus membranes.
Vitamin B-complex	100 mg daily	Contributes to healing of delicate skin and mucus membranes, especially when taken with vitamin A.
Vitamin C	500 mg three times daily	Powerful healing agent.
Zinc	15–30 mg daily	Good all-purpose healer.

What You Can Do

✓ Desist from scratching through underwear.
✓ Avoid citrus fruits and juices until healing is complete.
✓ Practice super hygiene (e.g. a warm bath a few hours before bed).
✓ Wear white underwear day and night to avoid skin-irritating dyes.
✓ Avoid long pajamas. Sleeping naked is best!
✓ Apply a nonprescription fungal cream if you suspect a fungal infection.
✓ Sprinkle a tablespoon of wheat germ on oatmeal, millet, or whole grain cereal daily until condition clears up.
✓ Add a tablespoon of brewer's yeast to a glass of tomato juice and drink daily until condition clears up.
✓ Eat foods high in vitamin A, including eggs, milk, cheese, cream, butter, yogurt, salmon, bass, halibut, mackerel, herring, whitefish, sardines, tuna, clams, shrimp, beef, chicken, pistachios, pecans, walnuts, lentils, and soybeans.
✓ Eat foods high in vitamin C, including rose hips, acerola cherries, guavas, black currants, red peppers, oranges, grapefruit and other citrus fruits, cabbage, papayas, cantaloupe, and tomatoes.
✓ Eat foods high in zinc, including seafood, sardines, oysters, soybeans, soy lecithin, kelp, legumes, meat, liver, eggs, brewer's yeast, mushrooms, poultry, whole grains, and pumpkin and sunflower seeds.

And Try This!

Try drinking a tablespoon of desiccated liver powder in freshly squeezed vegetable juice in the evening—an excellent source of B vitamins.

Did You Know?

For about a half century, doctors in Germany have used plain, unflavored, live culture yogurt to soothe rectal itch. It works for my patients. All you do is dip several thicknesses of facial tissue into a container of yogurt and spread it on the itching areas. Apply it before bedtime when it is least likely to rub off. Incidentally, plain Vaseline applied in the same way also helps the cause.

Raynaud's Disease

Raynaud's disease is an odd condition that causes the fingers and toes to become numb or tingle when exposed to cold temperatures. This can be an extreme such as going out into wintry weather or something trivial like entering an air-conditioned room, opening the refrigerator door, or even touching a glass containing a cold drink. Discovered in 1862 by Maurice Raynaud, a French physician, the disease is still not well understood by medical researchers.

Recognizing Raynaud's Disease

Raynaud's disease is more frequent in women than in men. Symptoms can include:

- White or blue fingers or toes
- Tingling in the fingers or toes
- Sores on fingers and toes and under nails
- Gangrene (usually only in extreme cases)

What Are the Causes of Raynaud's Disease?

The most that can be said about Raynaud's disease is that minute arteries (arterioles) overreact and go into spasms when extremities are exposed to cold. Oversensitive and overreactive nerves are thought to be the reason, although experts have not yet proven this to be the case. Factors that are believed to contribute to Raynaud's disease include the following:

- Stress
- Nutritional deficiencies
- Caffeine
- Drug reactions (especially to

- Low thyroid function
- Smoking

heart medications, migraine relievers, or decongestants)

What You Can Take

Nutrients

Name	Dosage	Benefits
Vitamin B-complex	100 mg daily	Helps break down carbohydrates and fats to release energy, and helps to bring about relaxation.
Vitamin E	400 IU daily	Promotes good circulation.
Chlorophyll	Two tablespoons daily	Promotes healing in sores that develop on fingers and toes and also enhances circulation.
Coenzyme Q-10	50 mg twice daily	Useful for making sure tissues are properly infused with oxygen.
Ginkgo biloba	60 mg twice daily	Very effective for increasing blood flow throughout the body.
Inositol-hexaniacinate (a nonflush form of niacin)	500 mg twice daily	Promotes good circulation.
Magnesium	500 mg daily	Relaxes constricted nerves and is highly effective against the condition.

Homeopathy

Name	Dosage	Benefits
Carbo vegetabilis	6c every hour up to six times daily until symptoms recede or disappear.	Helps relieve bluish colors and numbness in the extremities.

What You Can Do

✓ Give your fingers and toes a 2- or 3-minute topical massage with evening primrose oil or borage oil for relief.

✓ Don't smoke.

✓ Avoid caffeine.

✓ Test for low thyroid function (*see* HYPOTHYROIDISM).

✓ Avoid exposing hands and feet to cold.

✓ Eat foods high in vitamin E, including sunflower seeds, whole wheat, peanuts, cashews, almonds, walnuts, corn oil, soy oil, soy lecithin, spinach, asparagus, broccoli, and avocados.

✓ Eat foods high in magnesium, including blackstrap molasses, sunflower seeds, wheat germ, almonds, hazelnuts, Brazil nuts, pecans, walnuts, soybeans, soy lecithin, oats, barley, salmon, corn, avocados, bananas, cheese, tuna, and potatoes.

And Try This!

Try doing giant arm circles as fast as you can, rotating directions between both forward and backward. This can relieve symptoms by improving blood flow to the fingers.

Did You Know?

Two homeopathic remedies for this condition often help my patients when they can't get relief from other natural products: Arsenicum album 6c taken every half hour for four hours or Pulsatilla 6c taken at the same intervals for four hours. Arsenicum album is particularly effective when swelling in the fingers and toes accompanies feeling cold. Pulsatilla works best when applied warmth makes the fingers more uncomfortable.

Restless Leg Syndrome

What's in a name? If ever a medical term was self-explanatory, it is in the case of restless leg syndrome (RLS)—a condition where legs twitch or jerk involuntarily, and one suffered by millions. RLS is especially a problem at night since it can result in insomnia.

Recognizing Restless Leg Syndrome

- Irresistible urge to move legs
- Inability to sit or sleep for long without having to get up and walk
- A creeping sensation in the legs
- Numbness in the legs
- Exhaustion (from poor sleep due to RLS)

What Are the Causes of Restless Leg Syndrome?

- Nutritional deficiencies (especially folic acid and iron)
- Caffeine
- Stress
- Anxiety

What You Can Take

Nutrients

Name	Dosage	Benefits
Vitamin B-complex	100 mg daily	Necessary for maintaining the biochemical balance of all B vitamins when supplementing with any single B vitamin individually (like folic acid).
Vitamin E	400 IU daily for two months	Relieves symptoms of RLS.
Calcium	1,500 mg daily	Works well against RLS when taken together with magnesium and potassium.

Name	Dosage	Benefits
Folic acid	5 mg three times daily if deficient in folic acid *Warning:* Do not take this amount unless approved by a nutrition-oriented physician. 400 mcg daily has also been shown to be effective.	Deficiencies linked to RLS.
Magnesium	750 mg daily (250 mg after each meal)	Works well against RLS when taken together with calcium and potassium.
Potassium	99 mg before bedtime	Works well against RLS when taken together with magnesium and calcium.

Homeopathy

Name	Dosage	Benefits
Aconitie	6c twice daily	Most effective when RLS is triggered by stress.
Zincum metallicum	6c three times daily for a week to ten days	Helpful for those exhausted from many night risings and exceptionally restless legs.

What You Can Do

✓ Avoid caffeine.
✓ Work to relieve stress (*see* STRESS).
✓ Eat foods high in iron, including kidney, liver, eggs, millet, lentils, walnuts, oats, wheat, beef, buckwheat, and barley.
✓ Do not take supplemental iron without first consulting with a physician.
✓ Eat foods high in folic acid, including whole grains, wheat germ, bran, brown rice, liver, milk, beef, barley, chicken, tuna, salmon, lentils, legumes, brewer's yeast, cheese, oranges, mushrooms, and green leafy vegetables.
✓ Eat foods high in vitamin E, including sunflower seeds, whole wheat, peanuts, cashews, almonds, walnuts, corn oil,

soy oil, soy lecithin, spinach, asparagus, broccoli, butter oats, and avocados.

✓ Eat foods high in calcium, including buttermilk, yogurt (low fat), cheddar, parmesan and romano cheeses, carob, brewer's yeast, kale, kelp, broccoli, amaranth, teff, sesame seeds, and sardines.

✓ Eat foods high in magnesium, including blackstrap molasses, sunflower seeds, wheat germ, almonds, hazelnuts, Brazil nuts, pecans, walnuts, soybeans, soy lecithin, oats, barley, salmon, corn, avocados, bananas, cheese, tuna, and potatoes.

✓ Eat foods high in potassium, including bananas, cantaloupe, broccoli, avocados, Brussels sprouts, cauliflower, blackstrap molasses, brewer's yeast, brown rice, potatoes, legumes, dates, and whole grains.

And Try This!

Try running a vibrator over your legs for 5–10 minutes. This has helped some of my patients. Vibration seems to cause a release of endorphins, which not only kill pain but may also discourage RLS.

Did You Know?

In a study by biochemists S. Ayres and R. Mihan published in the *Journal of Applied Nutrition,* 7 of 9 patients were totally relieved of RLS on 400 IU daily of vitamin E for 2 months. The other two showed moderate improvement.

Rosacea (Patches of Red Skin)

Rosacea is a serious skin condition affecting the face that can resemble a bad case of acne. Unlike acne, however, it occurs most often in those of middle or later age. Rosacea is three times more common in women then men. But in men who develop rosacea, it tends to be more severe. Rosacea is not considered a serious threat to health, but is often unattractive and can lead to permanent cosmetic damage if left untreated.

Recognizing Rosacea

- Red and inflamed patches of facial skin
- Redness increases as disorder gets worse
- Sometimes a ruddy network of arteries that shows just under the skin
- Burning or swollen eyes

What Are the Causes of Rosacea?

- Poor digestion (lack of hydrochloric acid in the stomach)
- Lack of the pancreatic enzyme lipase
- Nutritional deficiencies (especially vitamins B_2 and A)
- Food and environmental allergies
- Local infection
- Menopausal flushing
- Smoking
- Alcohol
- Coffee
- Spicy foods
- Ginkgo biloba
- Stress

What You Can Take

Nutrients

Name	Dosage	Benefits
Vitamin A	10,000 IU daily	Effective against skin and mucus membrane ailments.
Vitamin B_2	50 mg daily	Deficiencies have been linked to rosacea.
Vitamin C	1,000 mg three times daily	Promotes the making of collagen that contributes to healthy membranes lining blood vessels and limits the release of histamine in allergic reaction.
Hydrochloric acid	Formula consisting of 648 mg of betaine hydrochloride and 130 mg of pepsin	Improves poor digestion. Deficiencies have been linked to rosacea.
Lipase (pancreatic enzyme)	1,400 mg of the pancreatic complex lipase, trypsin, and amylase	Deficiencies have been linked to rosacea.

| Zinc | 15–30 mg daily | Effective against rosacea, especially when taken with vitamin A. |

What You Can Do

✓ Avoid foods and supplements that cause capillary expansion and facial flushing, including niacin (vitamin B_3), ginkgo biloba, coffee, alcohol, and spicy foods.

✓ Avoid hot drinks in general.

✓ Work to relieve stress (*see* STRESS).

✓ Drink at least 8–10 glasses of pure spring water daily.

✓ Eat plenty of fresh fruits and vegetables.

✓ Test for food and environmental allergies (*see* ALLERGIES).

✓ Limit use of makeup.

✓ Eat foods high in vitamin A, including eggs, milk, cheese, cream, butter, yogurt, salmon, bass, halibut, mackerel, herring, whitefish, sardines, tuna, clams, shrimp, beef, chicken, pistachios, pecans, walnuts, lentils, and soybeans.

✓ Eat foods high in vitamin B_2, including brewer's yeast, alfalfa, spinach, liver, royal jelly, bee pollen, almonds, wheat germ, eggs, cheese, millet, chicken, mushrooms, soybeans, sunflower seeds, lamb, peas, blackstrap molasses, cottage cheese, sesame seeds, lentils, whole rye, turkey, and broccoli.

✓ Eat foods high in vitamin C, including rose hips, acerola cherries, guavas, black currants, red peppers, oranges, grapefruit and other citrus fruits, cabbage, papayas, cantaloupe, and tomatoes.

✓ Eat foods high in zinc, including seafood, sardines, oysters, soybeans, soy lecithin, kelp, legumes, meat, liver, eggs, brewer's yeast, mushrooms, poultry, whole grains, and pumpkin and sunflower seeds.

And Try This!

Try gently applying a natural aloe vera gel to areas of the face affected by rosacea. Aloe is universally recognized for its powerful healing properties, especially with respect to skin conditions.

Did You Know?

An interesting experiment reveals that vitamin B_2 can be critical to preventing and controlling rosacea. On the basis that a tiny mite called Demodex follicorum is thought to cause some cases of rosacea, researchers J. Johnson and R. Eckhardt, writing in *Archives of Ophthalmology,* implanted the skin of two groups of rats with these mites. Rats deficient in vitamin B_2 became infected, showing signs similar to rosacea in human beings. However, those adequately supplied with this vitamin rejected the mites.

Scurvy

A commonly held belief is that the disease scurvy, caused by a deficiency of vitamin C, is a thing of the past. This couldn't be more wrong, as expressed many times by the late Dr. Albert Szent Gyorgyi, who won the Nobel Prize for identifying vitamin C. There was total agreement from Nobel Laureate Dr. Linus Pauling, the most prominent vitamin C researcher in the last half of the twentieth century. True enough, today's scurvy is not as severe as that experienced by sailors of the seventeenth and eighteenth century. But scurvy isn't just a matter for medical historians yet either.

Recognizing Scurvy

Early signs of subclinical scurvy may include the following:

- Swollen and bleeding gums
- Tiny red blotches under the skin
- Tendency to bruise easily
- Low energy
- Wounds that won't heal
- Water retention
- Joint pains

What Are the Causes of Scurvy?

Scurvy is a disease caused by a deficiency of vitamin C. Factors that can contribute to inadequate levels of vitamin C in the body include the following:

* Not eating enough foods containing vitamin C
* Smoking
* Stress
* Aging
* Surgery
* Bacterial and viral infections
* Poor digestion
* Drug use
* Alcohol
* Environmental pollution

What You Can Take

Nutrients

Name	Dosage	Benefits
Vitamin C	500 mg three times daily	Prevents and can reverse scurvy.
Flavonoids	500 to 1,000 mg daily	Augments vitamin C in preventing and reversing scurvy.

What You Can Do

✓ Eat foods high in vitamin C, including rose hips, acerola cherries, guavas, black currants, red peppers, oranges, grapefruit and other citrus fruits, cabbage, papayas, cantaloupe, green vegetables, and tomatoes.
✓ Don't smoke.
✓ Avoid alcohol and drugs.
✓ Work to relieve stress (*see* STRESS).

And Try This!

Go for color when you buy vegetables and fruit, and you'll gain more vitamin C to prevent scurvy, plus flavonoids and antioxidants. Buy the greenest lettuce and other leafy veggies; the reddest tomatoes—they also contain more lycopene—red, rather than green or white grapes; red and yellow onions, rather than white (the former are richer in quercetin, a powerful antioxidant and antibacterial and antiviral substance).

Did You Know?

Recommended daily amounts of vitamin C may fall woefully short for most individuals. In his monumental book, *The Healing Factor: Vitamin C Against Disease*, Irwin Stone states that, for full correction of subclinical scurvy, a person weighing about 150 pounds should take in between 2,000 and 4,000 mg of vitamin C daily. Stone indicates that stress can skyrocket the daily requirement for vitamin C to about 15,000 mg daily, and that it is difficult, if not impossible, to supply one's needs for vitamin C only from foods.

Shingles (Herpes Zoster)

Many people who have had chicken pox as a child develop shingles (herpes zoster) during their adult life—usually past middle age. An infection of major spinal nerves that describe a semicircle around the body, shingles can causes a rash of small, round, fluid-filled blisters on one or both sides of the chest, and then if it progresses, excruciating neuralgic pain. The return of chicken pox in the form of shingles—both ailments are caused by the same virus—results from a weak immune system response.

Recognizing Shingles

- Rash of small, round, fluid-filled blisters on one or both sides of the chest
- Extreme itching
- Neuralgic pain
- Numbness
- Headache
- Fatigue

What Are the Causes of Shingles?

The underlying source of shingles is the varicella zoster virus, but breakouts result from an immune system too weak to keep the virus at bay. Many factors can weaken the immune system, including the following:

- Stress
- Poor nutrition
- Lack of sleep
- Environmental pollutants
- Food and environmental allergies
- Radiation or chemotherapy
- Enduring illness
- Aging
- Smoking
- Drug and alcohol use

What You Can Take

Nutrients

Name	Dosage	Benefits
Vitamin A	10,000 IU daily	Boosts immune function and accelerates healing of vesicles.
Vitamin B_{12}	1,000 mcg under the tongue daily	Contributes to nerve tissue metabolism.
Vitamin C	500 mg three times daily	Clears up rash and relieves pain associated with shingles.
Vitamin E	400–800 IU daily	Potent pain reliever.
Zinc	15–30 mg daily	Speeds up healing, especially when taken with vitamin A.

What You Can Do

✓ Keep in mind that although shingles can't be cured, it can be kept under control.

✓ Don't smoke.

✓ Avoid alcohol and drugs.

✓ Avoid sugar and refined carbohydrates (especially white flour).

✓ Avoid prescription medications where possible.

✓ Add a piece of fresh fruit or vegetable to every meal.

✓ Get plenty of sleep.

✓ Drink at least 8–10 glasses of pure spring water daily.

✓ Work to relieve stress (*see* STRESS).

✓ Test for food and environmental allergies (*see* ALLERGIES).

✓ Eat foods high in vitamin A, including eggs, milk, cheese, cream, butter, yogurt, salmon, bass, halibut, mackerel, herring, whitefish, sardines, tuna, clams, shrimp, beef, chicken, pistachios, pecans, walnuts, lentils, and soybeans.

✓ Eat foods high in vitamin C, including rose hips, acerola cherries, guavas, black currants, red peppers, oranges, grapefruit and other citrus fruits, cabbage, papayas, cantaloupe, and tomatoes.

✓ Eat foods high in vitamin E, including sunflower seeds, whole wheat, peanuts, cashews, almonds, walnuts, corn oil, soy oil, soy lecithin, spinach, asparagus, broccoli, oats, and avocados.

✓ Eat foods high in zinc, including seafood, sardines, oysters, soybeans, soy lecithin, kelp, legumes, meat, liver, eggs, brewer's yeast, mushrooms, poultry, whole grains, and pumpkin and sunflower seeds.

And Try This!

Try applying the following topical application to rash areas: zinc oxide, a tablespoon of aloe vera juice or gel, and the contents of two 400 IU vitamin E capsules. It brings welcome itch or pain relief within an hour and promotes healing.

Did You Know?

The late Dr. Fred Klenner, pioneer researcher with vitamin C, cleared up painful cases of shingles within 3 days. In an experimental study, Dr. Klenner injected 8 herpes zoster patients with 2,000–3,000 mg of vitamin C every 12 hours, and also had them take 1,000 mg orally every 2 hours. Seven patients were overjoyed to report that their pain dissipated 2 hours after their initial injection. The eighth patient, a diabetic, required 14 injections, but he was free of the rash and all pain within 2 weeks.

Sinusitis

The sinuses are hollow, mucus-lined cavities that warm and humidify the air we breathe and flush out irritating, harmful dust and pollens. There are four pairs of sinuses—two above the eyes, two below the eyes, two just above the bridge of the nose, and two set deep in the skull. On the bottom of them, tiny openings a little larger than the point of a ballpoint pen release mucus into channels that empty into the nasal cavity. Trouble starts when the sinuses become inflamed from allergies, colds, bacterial and viral infections, or an overgrowth of fungus. Swelling causes the tiny openings to close. Then mucus thickens and collects, serving as an ideal environment for bacteria to multiply. And guess what? You've got sinusitis.

Recognizing Sinusitis

- Headaches
- Earaches
- Sinus pressure
- A fetid odor sensed in the nostrils
- Poor sense of smell
- Coughs
- Post nasal drip
- Difficulty breathing
- Fever

What Are the Causes of Sinusitis?

- Food and environmental allergies (especially dairy products)
- Colds
- Bacterial and viral infections
- Fungal overgrowths
- Injury to the nose
- Smoking
- Weak immune system

What You Can Take

Nutrients

Name	Dosage	Benefits
Vitamin A	25,000 IU daily *Warning:* Pregnant or pregnancy-eligible women should take no more than 10,000 IU daily.	Immune booster that helps prevent sinusitis.
Bioflavonoids	500 mg and 200 mg of vitamin C every two hours	Reduces histamines without the side effects of antihistamine medications.
Omega-3 fatty acids	300 mg of EPA and 200 mg of DHA three times daily	Reduces histamines without the side effects of antihistamine medications.
Zinc	30 mg daily	Immune booster that helps prevent sinusitis, especially when taken with vitamin A.

Herbs

Name	Dosage	Benefits
Astragalus	200 mg three times daily	Strengthens immune system.
Cat's claw	250 mg twice daily	Strengthens immune system.
Echinacea	200 mg three times daily	Strengthens immune system.
Goldenseal with bromelain	250 mg of each every three hours	Strengthens immune system.

Name	Dosage	Benefits
Maitake (mushroom)	200 mg twice daily	Strengthens immune system.
Reishi (mushroom)	500 mg twice daily *Warning:* Not to be taken with an anti-coagulant.	Strengthens immune system.

What You Can Do

✓ Test for food and environmental allergies (*see* ALLERGIES).
✓ Avoid environmental triggers for sinusitis such as smog, auto exhaust, cigarette smoke, and chlorine fumes.
✓ Avoid food triggers for sinusitis such as beef, citrus fruits, clams, dairy products, eggs, lobster, oysters, peanuts, pork, shrimp, soy, sugar, wheat products, and additives in processed foods.
✓ Don't smoke.
✓ Remember that antihistamine for sinusitis can cause side effects.
✓ Breathe steam from hot water with a towel tent overhead for relief.
✓ Add two or three drops of eucalyptus or peppermint oil to hot water for help in breathing.
✓ Open nasal passages with fumes from freshly cut onions or ground horseradish.
✓ Get plenty of rest.
✓ Drink at least 8–10 glasses of pure spring water daily.
✓ Use care when blowing nose (don't blow too hard).
✓ See your doctor if you discharge blood from your nose.

And Try This!

Try one of the prime homeopathic remedies for opening stubborn sinus passages: nux vomica. My patients have experienced relief taking two 6X or 30X pellets of this formula every 3 hours.

Did You Know?

Decongestants are addictive, raise blood pressure, and can cause a worsening of the exact conditions they are supposed to treat once you stop using them.

Spina Bifida

It is critically important to correct misunderstandings about folic acid and its ability to protect fetuses from spina bifida, complications of incomplete closing of the neural tube. Too little knowledge can lead to errors in intake and supplementation of this B vitamin with serious consequences to the fetus and the mother-to-be. These errors can range from the appropriate stage in pregnancy when folic acid supplementation should be started to how much should be taken and when.

Recognizing Spina Bifida

Spina bifida occurs in only 1-2 cases per 30,000, but the odds increase to 1 in 30 for women who have already given birth to a spina bifida infant. In affected infants, the lower part of the neural tube may fail to develop normally and to close. It then remains open until birth, leaving sensitive nerves exposed. Nerve damage can cause paralysis and an inability to control bowel and bladder, and sometimes, a larger-than-normal skull and water retention, compressing the brain.

What Are the Causes of Spina Bifida?

Spina bifida results from a deficiency of folic acid in the mother as early as the time of conception. Without sufficient folic acid, damage can begin by the fourth week of pregnancy.

What You Can Take

Nutrients

Name	Dosage	Benefits
Folic acid	400 mcg following both breakfast and dinner	Deficiencies are the direct cause of spina bifida.
Vitamin B-complex	100 mg daily	Necessary for maintaining the biochemical balance of all B vitamins when supplementing with any single B vitamin individually.
Vitamin B$_{12}$	1,000 mcg under the tongue daily	Essential when supplementing with folic acid, as folic acid can mask symptoms of pernicious anemia, which is caused by a lack of vitamin B$_{12}$.
Vitamin E	400–800 IU daily	Deficiencies linked to spina bifida and other neural tube defects.
Lecithin	Two 1200 mg capsules or 2 tsp of granules twice daily	Contributes to the soundness of the nerves in the womb, which is essential for preventing spina bifida.

What You Can Do

✓ Prepare for pregnancy now (with proper supplementation) because you can never know exactly when it will take place.

✓ Remember that the most critical time for the fetus is the first trimester, and too little folic acid intake can lead to spina bifida and brain abnormalities.

✓ Avoid alcohol and soft drinks.

✓ Avoid sugar and other refined carbohydrates.

✓ Protect the fetus with at least 60 grams or protein daily, a fresh fruit or vegetable with every meal, and a green salad daily.

✓ Eat foods high in folic acid, including beef, green leafy veg-

etables, beans, lentils, whole grains, liver, milk, mushrooms, oranges, tuna, and salmon.
✓ Eat foods high in vitamin E, including sunflower seeds,
whole wheat, peanuts, cashews, almonds, walnuts, corn oil,
soy oil, soy lecithin, spinach, asparagus, broccoli, butter
oats, and avocados.
✓ Eat foods high in calcium, including buttermilk, milk, yogurt (low fat), cheddar, parmesan and romano cheeses,
carob, brewer's yeast, kale, kelp, broccoli, amaranth, teff, almonds, sesame seeds, and sardines.

And Try This!

*Try two 1,200 mg capsules of lecithin daily, especially if
you're hoping to have a baby. A little-known fact about
this nutrient—which is found in soybeans, eggs, liver and
wheat germ—is that it helps to prevent spina bifida. The
granular form—also two teaspoons daily—works as well.
You may want to avoid the gooey, fluid form, however,
because it stubbornly sticks to the teeth.*

Did You Know?

Dr. Michael Laurence and his team at the Welsh National
School of Medicine conducted three separate studies on neural
tube damage that produced the following results:

1. All spina bifida cases occurred in women on poor diets in
   the first trimester, the period during which the delicate
   neural tube is forming and most susceptible to damage.
2. In the second study, spina bifida cases again were traced to
   poor diet. Sisters who had no history of spina bifida births
   and those who had were compared. The latter group had
   poor-quality diets—particularly in the first trimester. Sisters
   in the first group, on a good diet, were upset that their sisters
   practically lived on processed convenience food.
3. The third study focused on intake of folic acid and found it
   to be the most important anti–spina bifida nutrient of all.

Stress

Stress is an insidious ailment. Simply defined, it refers to a reaction to any event that upsets normal physical or psychological functioning. As it steals nutrients, stress can cause a multitude of disorders, including cancer, liver disease, dental cavities, menstrual irregularities, high blood pressure, low blood sugar, sleeplessness, adrenal exhaustion, and even outbreaks on the skin. Numerous studies reveal that emotional stressors such as the loss of a mate, chronic worrying, hostility, and anger can contribute to heart disease and often death. Estimates are that as much as 80 percent of all the health problems currently suffered by Americans can be linked to stress.

Recognizing Stress

Stress can be hard to detect in its own right because the effects usually take the form of more categorical types of conditions such as those mentioned above. For example, someone overwhelmed at work may not be able to sleep at night. Is she suffering from insomnia or a bad case of stress? The answer is both. So, aside from the general feeling of "being stressed out" that most of us are familiar with, are there certain stress symptoms? Such a list would be endless, but those at the top would include the following:

- Anxiety
- Irritability
- Depression
- Fatigue
- High blood pressure
- Stomach problems
- Insomnia
- Headaches
- Appetite changes
- Grinding of teeth (bruxism)
- Trouble breathing
- Lack of sexual desire

What Are the Causes of Stress?

Stress is a highly personal matter, in that we all react to certain things, both physical and psychological things, differently. Studies point to the following life events as some of the most universally stressful:

- Death of a family member or loved one
- Divorce
- Loss of job or serious trouble at work
- Serious illness or injury to a family member or loved one
- New marriage
- New job
- Moving to a new residence
- Birth of a child
- Child leaving home for the first time
- Sexual problems
- Financial trouble
- Holidays
- Vacations
- Drug and/or alcohol abuse

What You Can Take

Nutrients

Name	Dosage	Benefits
Vitamin B-complex	100 mg daily	Necessary for maintaining the biochemical balance of all B vitamins when supplementing with any single B vitamin individually.
Vitamin B$_2$	100 mg daily	Protects the nervous system from the harmful effects of stress.
Vitamin C	500 mg three times daily	Rebalances adrenal glands that become exhausted due to stress.
Vitamin D	400 IU daily	Relaxant effects useful against stress.
Calcium citrate	1,000 mg daily	Deficiencies occur due to stress, resulting in nervous disorders.
5-HTP	100 mg thirty minutes before bedtime daily	Promotes good sleep.
Magnesium	500 mg daily	Deficiencies occur due to stress, resulting in nervous disorders.
Melatonin	1–3 mg before bedtime daily	Promotes good sleep.
Zinc	30 mg daily	Protects immune system from the effects of stress.

Herbs

Name	Dosage	Benefits
Kava	250 mg daily	Relaxant that promotes good sleep.
Valerian (powdered)	200 mg thirty minutes before going to bed daily	Widely recognized for its positive effects on sleep.

What You Can Do

✓ Exercise daily.
✓ Get plenty of sleep.
✓ Don't smoke.
✓ Avoid alcohol, drugs, and caffeine.
✓ Avoid sugar and other refined carbohydrates.
✓ Purge negative emotions, pent-up anger, hostilities, and worry to avoid cardiovascular disorders.
✓ Rid yourself of fears, anxieties, and hatred with the help of a spouse, a friend, priest, minister, or rabbi.
✓ Do a favor for someone else that takes time and effort in order to get your mind off yourself.
✓ Try to get 100 laughs a day for relief of tension.
✓ Cry in private to rid yourself of frustration and stress.
✓ Eat a high-protein diet, including meat, poultry, eggs, and fish.
✓ Eat foods high in vitamin B_2, including brewer's yeast, alfalfa, spinach, liver, royal jelly, bee pollen, almonds, wheat germ, eggs, cheese, millet, chicken, mushrooms, soybeans, sunflower seeds, lamb, peas, blackstrap molasses, cottage cheese, sesame seeds, lentils, whole rye, turkey, and broccoli.
✓ Eat foods high in vitamin C, including rose hips, acerola cherries, guavas, black currants, red peppers, oranges, grapefruit and other citrus fruits, cabbage, papayas, cantaloupe, and tomatoes.
✓ Eat foods high in vitamin D, including cod liver oil, eggs, herring, organ meats, salmon, and sardines.
✓ Eat foods high in magnesium, including blackstrap molasses, sunflower seeds, wheat germ, almonds, hazelnuts, Brazil nuts, pecans, walnuts, soybeans, soy lecithin, oats,

barley, salmon, corn, avocados, bananas, cheese, tuna, and potatoes.

✓ Eat foods high in zinc, including seafood, sardines, oysters, soybeans, soy lecithin, kelp, legumes, meat, liver, eggs, brewer's yeast, mushrooms, poultry, whole grains, and pumpkin and sunflower seeds.

✓ Remember and repeat the Bible quotation: "A merry heart doeth good like a medicine."

And Try This!

Try using the Benson relaxing technique: Inhale deeply for ten counts, then release it slowly for twelve counts while murmuring the word "one."

Did You Know?

A study by Swedish researchers I. Liljefors and R. H. Rahe reported in *Psychosomatic Medicine* produced surprising results concerning the destructive power of stress. Investigating adult, male, identical twins, they discovered in each pair that the twin more dissatisfied with experiences in childhood, educational level, and life achievements had a significant additional amount of severe coronary artery disease. Being dissatisfied with life was a far more powerful determinant than high cholesterol, high blood pressure, or obesity.

Stretch Marks

After giving birth, it is not unusual for women to develop long, wavy, seam-like stretch marks on the skin of their bellies. It is not unusual for heavy women who have lost much weight to have stretch marks on their bellies, breasts, and thighs. However, it *is* unusual for normal weight young women who have not been pregnant or overweight to develop stretch marks. Yet more and more of them come to dermatologists in tears, embarrassed by blemishes that seem to have no immediate explanation.

Recognizing Stretch Marks

Stretch marks can most often be found on the bellies, buttocks, breasts, and thighs. They are usually red when they first appear and may eventually turn white.

What Are the Causes of Stretch Marks?

Stretch marks occur as the result of extreme skin stress that causes underlying tissue fibers to tear. Contributing factors may include:

- Pregnancy
- Rapid weight gain and/or loss
- Crash diets
- Subnormal diet (enough calories but not enough nourishment)
- Lack of regular exercise
- Excessive sun exposure
- Diabetes
- Low thyroid function

What You Can Take

Nutrients

Name	Dosage	Benefits
Vitamin A	25,000 IU daily *Warning:* Pregnant or pregnancy-eligible women should take no more than 10,000 IU daily.	Important to integrity of the skin and underlying tissue, and to the body's ability to use protein.
Vitamin B-complex	100 mg daily	Necessary for maintaining the biochemical balance of all B vitamins when supplementing with any single B vitamin.
Vitamin B_5	300 mg daily	Helps prevent dermis tears and stretch marks.
Vitamin C	500 mg three times daily	Essential for strong and resilient connective tissue.

Name	Dosage	Benefits
Vitamin E	400–800 IU daily	Helps the body utilize vitamin A and protects cell membranes from damage.
Silica	11 mg daily	Protects against injuries that cause stretch marks.
Zinc	30 mg daily	Protects against injuries that cause stretch marks.

Herbs

Name	Dosage	Benefits
Horsetail	440 mg daily	A rich source of silica.

What You Can Do

✓ Exercise daily.

✓ Maintain a health body weight (see OVERWEIGHT).

✓ Avoid crash diets.

✓ Avoid excessive sun exposure.

✓ Avoid processed foods.

✓ Avoid sugar and other refined carbohydrates.

✓ Drink at least 8–10 glasses of pure spring water daily.

✓ Eat a diet high in protein, including eggs, meat, fish, poultry, and dairy products. Alternative protein sources for vegetarians include fruits, vegetables, grains, legumes, nuts, and seeds.

✓ Eat foods high in silica, including vegetables, whole grains, and seafood.

✓ Eat foods high in vitamin A, including eggs, milk, cheese, cream, butter, yogurt, salmon, bass, halibut, mackerel, herring, whitefish, sardines, tuna, clams, shrimp, beef, chicken, pistachios, pecans, walnuts, lentils, and soybeans.

✓ Eat foods high in vitamin C, including rose hips, acerola cherries, guavas, black currants, red peppers, oranges, grapefruit and other citrus fruits, cabbage, papayas, cantaloupe, and tomatoes.

✓ Eat foods high in vitamin E, including sunflower seeds, whole wheat, peanuts, cashews, almonds, walnuts, corn oil, soy oil, soy lecithin, spinach, asparagus, broccoli, oats, and avocados.

And Try This!

Try massaging a combination of aloe vera juice (2 table-spoons) and the contents of 400 IU of natural vitamin E mixed together into stretch marks before bedtime and in the morning. Aloe vera is noted for penetrating the skin deeply to heal wounds and burns.

Did You Know?

During a medical conference, the late and eminent bio-chemist Carl C. Pfeiffer, Director of Princeton's Brain Bio Center, told me that males new to weight lifting sometimes develop stretch marks. Dr. Pfeiffer relayed the case of a young man in poor health who wanted to build his health by weight lifting. He tried to do too much too fast. When he lifted a heavy weight, he could actually feel his underskin (dermis) tearing. His stretch marks showed in the skin of his shoulder girdle. Relative to an overweight condition, men can also develop belly stretch marks when they lose poundage, but not in as great numbers as women.

Stroke

Stroke refers to a cut-off of oxygenated blood to the brain that suffocates and kills brain cells, causing a loss of speech or coordination, paralysis, or even death. Always considered a serious and extensive problem, strokes are even more numerous than previously estimated. According to a survey reported in the *Medical Tribune,* the annual number of strokes in the United States is 50 percent higher than previously estimated—750,000, instead of 500,000. Other enlightening statistics from this study disclose that almost 30 percent of all stroke victims had had previous strokes. This figure soared to 50 percent for patients over 75. Twelve percent of all stroke victims die in the hospital.

Recognizing Stroke

Like an early warning system that detects an invading missile, early warning signs frequently precede a stroke. Symptoms can include:

- Fainting
- Dizziness
- Unexplained weakness
- Blurred vision
- Disorientation
- Hearing loss
- Numbness
- Difficulty speaking
- Partial paralysis

Warning: Contact your doctor or get to a hospital immediately at the first sign of stroke.

What Are the Causes of Stroke?

Eighty percent of strokes are caused by abnormal blood clotting. Conditions responsible other than clots include blood-blocking plaque in the arteries, rupturing of arterial walls due to high blood pressure, and capillary fragility that permits bleeding and consequent excessive pressure on sensitive brain cells. The most well-established risk factors for stroke include the following:

- Heart disease
- High blood pressure
- Elevated blood fats
- Stress
- Smoking
- Alcohol
- Diabetes
- Overweight
- Diet high in salt

What You Can Take

Nutrients

Name	Dosage	Benefits
Vitamin C	1,000 mg with 500 mg of bioflavonoid three times daily	Strengthens fragile capillaries and keeps low-density lipoproteins (LDL) from oxidizing and adhering to capillary walls.
Acetyl-L-carnitine	1,500 mg daily	Helpful for recovering after a stroke has occurred.

Name	Dosage	Benefits
Grape seed or pine bark extract	100–300 mg daily	Antioxidant twenty times more powerful than vitamin C that corrects capillary fragility.

Herbs

Name	Dosage	Benefits
Guggulipid	50–100 mg twice daily	Reduces blood viscosity and protects against blood clots. Also reduces blood trigly-cerides and improves a poor HDL-LDL ratio.
Tylophora asthmatica	120 mg daily	A key Indian herb in Ayurvedic medicine that blocks the release of histamines and other inflammatories.

What You Can Do

✓ Eat foods that can help to prevent abnormal blood clotting leading to strokes, including garlic and onions, fish or omega-3 oil, red wine, tea, vegetables, hot chili pepper, black mushrooms, olive oil, cloves, cumin, ginger, and turmeric.

✓ Eat foods high in vitamin C and bioflavonoids, including oranges, apricots, blackberries, black currants, cherries, lemons, plums, green vegetables, and buckwheat.

✓ Don't smoke.

✓ Avoid alcohol.

✓ Avoid salt.

✓ Exercise daily.

✓ Maintain healthy body weight (see OVERWEIGHT).

✓ Work to relieve stress (see STRESS).

And Try This!

Try consulting with a physician trained in hyperbaric oxygen therapy—a treatment involving 100 percent oxygen administered by mask in a compressed air chamber that has proven highly effective in patients recovering from strokes.

Did You Know?

Dr. Jiang He, assistant professor of epidemiology at the Tulane University School of Public Health, studied the risk of stroke and heart attack to 9,000 individuals from age 25 to 74. Over a four-year period, intake of sodium (salt) was noted. Then volunteers were checked for strokes and heart attack six times over a 10-year period. Findings riveted attention on 2,699 overweight individuals who consumed 6 g of sodium or more daily. Thirty-two percent had an increased risk of stroke and an 89 percent increase in stroke-related death, a 44 percent increase in deaths caused by coronary artery-related death, a 61 percent increase in heart disease death, and a 39 percent increase in death from all causes. "This is the first study to identify a strong independent correlation between high sodium intake and stroke, heart attack, and mortality," wrote Dr. He.

Sunburn

Lying on the beach and burning until you're well done may cause more damage than you think due to a little known danger over and above skin cancer, made even more likely because of the thinning ozone layer. Sunburn can severely depress the immune system, making you more vulnerable to many infections and diseases.

Recognizing Sunburn

The average sunburn is a first-degree burn characterized by red skin that is hotter than normal and may be painful to touch. Once the initial inflammation has faded, the exposed area usually darkens to a tan, perhaps peeling eventually, but not always. Severe sunburns may also blister and be accompanied by swelling and more intense pain. Such symptoms point to a second-degree burn and may require the attention of a physician to guard against infection.

What Are the Causes of Sunburn?

Sunburn occurs due to an overexposure of the skin to ultraviolet rays produced by the sun. Individuals differ in their sensitivity to such exposure depending on skin type.

What You Can Take

Nutrients

Name	Dosage	Benefits
Vitamin C	500 mg three times daily	Promotes healing of damaged skin tissue.
Vitamin E	800 IU daily	Fights against free radicals brought on by sunburn.

What You Can Do

✓ Take a cold shower for 15 minutes, then spread on aloe vera gel to promote healing.

✓ Drink at least 8–10 glasses of pure spring water daily.

✓ Use a combination of one part olive oil and two parts of apple cider vinegar spread evenly on exposed skin.

✓ Guard your skin with topical vitamin C.

✓ Use the ointment or oil form of St. John's wort to soothe burns.

✓ Apply cold water to burns with a washcloth.

✓ Place the cooling juice of a cucumber on the burns with a washcloth.

✓ Wear protective clothing when spending significant amounts of time in the sun.

✓ Avoid further sun exposure until affected areas of the skin recover completely.

✓ Eat foods high in vitamin C, including rose hips, acerola cherries, guavas, black currants, red peppers, oranges, grapefruit and other citrus fruits, cabbage, papayas, cantaloupe, and tomatoes.

✓ Eat foods high in vitamin E, including sunflower seeds, whole wheat, peanuts, cashews, almonds, walnuts, corn oil, soy oil, soy lecithin, spinach, asparagus, broccoli, oats, and avocados.

And Try This!

Try spreading the following paste developed by a noted herbalist, the late Dr. John Christopher, on sunburned skin: half cup of honey, half cup of wheat germ oil, mixed with an equal amount of comfrey leaf or root. Then cover it lightly with gauze. The initial application should be left on with the next application spread over it the following day.

Did You Know?

A team of Australian researchers led by Dr. Peter Hersey, of Sydney Hospital, tested volunteers exposed to direct sunlight for 30 minutes a day for 12 days. Cells known to suppress immune system response increased and certain white cells that turn on immune system reaction decreased. A frightening aspect of this study was that these cells remained abnormal for 2 weeks after sunbathing had been discontinued. Dr. Hersey observed that his team's finding may explain how excessive sun exposure can cause skin cancer, and why so many people develop cold sores from herpes simplex virus after sunning.

Tinnitus (Ringing in the Ears)

One of the most ill-fitting names for a human ailment is tinnitus, Latin for "ringing in the ears." Why ill-fitting? Because the range of persisting sounds in the ears goes far beyond mere ringing: the buzzing of a bee, the beat of tom-toms, a Niagara Falls roar, the whir of a bandsaw, the hiss of steam, ticking, clacking, throbbing. Tinnitus patients usually drown out sounds that, according to some, drive them insane by boosting the volume on the stereo or TV. Some play music all night in order to sleep.

Recognizing Tinnitus

The main symptom of tinnitus is a continuous ringing, buzzing, or hissing in the ears, which can also be accompanied by pain.

What Are the Causes of Tinnitus?

Factors believed to cause or contribute to the onset of tinnitus include the following:

- Exposure to loud noises such as rock music or machinery
- Excessive earwax
- Inner ear infections
- Smoking
- Alcohol and/or drug use
- Caffeine
- Common medications such as aspirin and antibiotics
- Poor circulation
- Nutritional deficiencies

What You Can Take

Nutrients

Name	Dosage	Benefits
Vitamin A	10,000 IU daily	Good to take when supplementing with zinc.
Vitamin B-complex	100 mg daily	Necessary for maintaining the biochemical balance of all B vitamins when supplementing with any single B vitamin.
Vitamin B_6	50 mg three times daily	Aids in the formation of chemicals that both stimulate and regulate central nervous system and brain responses important to hearing.
Vitamin B_{12}	1,000 mcg under the tongue daily	Important to the production of myelin, the substance that insulates nerves.
Ginkgo biloba	60 mg twice daily	Increases blood circulation in the ears.

Magnesium	400 mg daily	Keeps arteries from constricting and limiting blood supply and nutrients essential to supporting nerve function, especially in the ears and brain.
Manganese	30 mg daily	Deficiencies can contribute to tinnitus.
Zinc	90 mg daily for fifteen days, then down to 30 mg and 2 mg of copper to retain proper zinc-copper ratio	Shown to produce good results in tinnitus patients.

What You Can Do

✓ Avoid extended exposure to loud noise.
✓ Avoid caffeine and alcohol.
✓ Don't smoke.
✓ Check for an excessive buildup of earwax or ear infections.
✓ Check with your doctor about possible side effects to any medications you may be taking.
✓ People who suffer from tinnitus often complain of vertigo and dizziness, both of which can be symptoms related to problems of the inner ear, the heart, or the brain. These people should see a doctor to rule out anemia, atherosclerosis, labyrinthitis, and hypertension as possible causes of the tinnitus.
✓ Cope with stress: stress aggravates tinnitus. Stress reduction techniques, such as Yoga, will help to eliminate tension and tinnitus.
✓ Eat foods high in vitamin A, including eggs, milk, cheese, cream, butter, yogurt, salmon, bass, halibut, mackerel, herring, whitefish, sardines, tuna, clams, shrimp, beef, chicken, pistachios, pecans, walnuts, lentils, and soybeans.
✓ Eat foods high in vitamin B_6, including brewer's yeast, brown rice, whole wheat, royal jelly, soybeans, rye, lentils, sunflower seeds, alfalfa, salmon, wheat germ, tuna, bran, walnuts, cashews, peanuts, peas, liver, avocados, beans, turkey, oats, chicken, halibut, lamb, and bananas.

✓ Eat foods high in vitamin B_{12}, including liver, sardines, mackerel, herring, red snapper, flounder, salmon, lamb, Swiss cheese, blue cheese, eggs, haddock, beef, halibut, anchovies, chicken, turkey, milk, and butter.

✓ Eat foods high in magnesium, including blackstrap molasses, sunflower seeds, wheat germ, almonds, hazelnuts, Brazil nuts, pecans, walnuts, soybeans, soy lecithin, oats, barley, salmon, corn, avocados, bananas, cheese, tuna, and potatoes.

✓ Eat foods high in zinc, including seafood, sardines, oysters, soybeans, soy lecithin, kelp, legumes, meat, liver, eggs, brewer's yeast, mushrooms, poultry, whole grains, and pumpkin and sunflower seeds.

And Try This!

The herb ginkgo biloba increases circulation in and around the ear area and is commonly used to treat tinnitus. Take two tablets of the standardized extract three times daily with meals.

Did You Know?

One interesting theory as to the cause of tinnitus is that some ears magnify sounds of the body's working: the thrust of blood through arteries and capillaries—especially those in the cochlea, the main organ of hearing that's shaped like a snail's shell and through a somewhat circulation-impaired carotid artery. Additional subtle but magnified sounds are thought to be continuous infinitesimal movements of cells, incessant ear muscle contractions, as well as hollow noises from an inflamed mucus membrane.

Ulcers

Ulcers of the stomach and duodenum, the fore part of the small intestine, are painful sores. Coping with them is a "don't do it yourself" project. Work closely with your alternative doctor.

Recognizing Ulcers

Gnawing pain in the stomach area before meals, an hour or more after, or during the night is a good indication of an ulcer. Food, antacids, or vomiting lessen or eliminate the pain. Tenderness of the abdominal area is a telltale symptom. Blood in waste matter or vomit and sudden, intense pain may signal ulcer perforation and internal bleeding. This may be a life-threatening emergency.

If you suspect an ulcer, have your doctor test you with an X-ray or the even more revealing endoscopic exam with a fiber-optic instrument.

What Are the Causes of Ulcers?

- Erosion of the protective mucus membrane in the stomach or duodenum by powerful digestive acids
- Helicobacter pylori bacteria that infects the stomach or intestinal wall, reducing the protection of the mucus membrane and permitting digestive juices to etch away tissue, a blood test can reveal such an infection
- Frequent long-term use of aspirins, ibuprofen, or other non-steroidal antiinflammatory drugs (NSAIDs)
- Poor diet
- Stress
- Smoking
- Alcohol
- Caffeine
- Processed foods
- Milk (to milk intolerants or those allergic)
- Allergies
- Gluten

What You Can Take

Nutrients

Name	Dosage	Benefits
Vitamin A	10,000 IU daily	Protects mucus membranes.
Vitamin C	500 mg three times daily	Blocks growth of H. pylori.
Gamma oryzanol	100 mg three times a day for thirty days	Promotes healing.
L-Glutamine	500 mg three times daily	Soothes, heals digestive tract cells.
Flavonoids	1,000 mg three times daily	Blocks growth of H. pylori and boosts immune system.
Zinc	30 mg daily	Teams with vitamin A to enhance healing.

Herbs

Name	Dosage	Benefits
Aloe vera	Half-cup of juice three times daily for thirty days	Acts to stop bleeding, lessens stomach acid secretions, and promotes healing.
Cabbage juice	⅕ quart five times daily	Enhances healing.
Deglycerrhizinated licorice (DGL)	Two chewable 250–500 mg tablets 15 to 30 minutes before meals and an hour before bedtime	Promotes health of stomach and intestinal lining.

What You Can Do

✓ Have your doctor verify the presence of ulcers.
✓ Get immediate treatment for bloody stools or vomit, usually indicative of a perforated ulcer.
✓ Take direction of an alternative doctor in coping with an ulcer.
✓ See ALLERGIES for methods to find offending foods and eliminate them.

✓ Stop smoking.

✓ Stop drinking alcohol.

✓ Eliminate caffeine-containing drinks: coffee, soft drinks, and chocolate.

✓ Eat foods rich in vitamin A or its predecessor, beta-carotene, including cod liver oil, beef liver, carrots, yams, watercress, red peppers, winter squash, egg yolks, apricots, fish, muscle meats. (Whole milk is vitamin A–rich. However, you may be milk-intolerant or allergic.)

✓ Eat vitamin C–rich foods and supplements, including rose hips, acerola cherries, guava, black currants red and green peppers, chives, strawberries, papaya, cantaloupe. loganberries, tomatoes, cabbage, and raspberries.

✓ Eat glutamine-containing foods, including meat, fish, beans, and peas.

✓ Eat flavonoids in foods: quercetin in yellow and red onions, red grapes, and apples; and rutin in buckwheat.

✓ Eat zinc-rich foods, including beef liver, dark meat, chicken and turkey, eggs, nuts, and wheat germ.

And Try This!

Increase your dietary protein. Protein-containing foods are rich in most of the vitamins and minerals suggested above, and they speed healing. Add fiber in fresh vegetables and fruit. Several studies show that fiber is helpful in coping with ulcers.

Did You Know?

Garnett Cheney, M.D., a Stanford University professor, discovered the cabbage juice treatment for ulcers. Thirteen of his ulcer patients were given a fifth of a quart of freshly squeezed cabbage juice five times daily, and every one of them was healed after 7.3 to 10.4 days. Dr. Cheney named cabbage juice vitamin U, because it reduced ulcers to the past tense.

Uterine Fibroids

A wave of fear engulfed Daphne. It was nowhere near her period time, yet she felt a gush of blood that started to seep through her clothing. She worried about this hemorrhaging until her gynecologist examined her and assured her that "in all probability, you have uterine fibroids that are benign." At least half of the women between ages 35 and 40 have anywhere from one to dozens of fibroids, he told her.

Recognizing Uterine Fibroids

Symptoms:

- Bleeding at the wrong time of the month
- Excessive bleeding during periods
- Pain in the bladder and bowels as a fibroid presses on a pelvic nerve
- Frequent urination
- Constipation
- Lower back pain

What Are the Causes of Uterine Fibroids?

- An inherited tendency
- Excessive estrogen secretion
- Excess weight
- High-fat diet
- Alcohol
- Deficiency of B-complex vitamins

What You Can Take?

Nutrients

Name	Dosage	Benefits
Vitamin B-complex	50–100 mg daily	Detoxifies excess estrogen, which creates a greater need for these nutrients.
Magnesium	400 mg daily	Detoxifies estrogen.
Probiotics	Up to 20 billion cells	Makes liver able to detoxify

| (including acidophilus) | daily | estrogen. |

Herbs

Name	Dosage	Benefits
Borage oil	500 mg twice daily	Works with Shepherd's purse, to reduce bleeding.
Chasteberry (also called Vitex)	225 mg daily	Helps balance hormone relationships; slows fibroid growth.
Shepherd's purse	50 drops three times daily	Works with borage oil to decrease bleeding.

What You Can Do

✓ Try to keep fibroids from growing out of control, because they have the potential of causing infertility or a miscarriage and, possibly, necessitate a hysterectomy.

✓ Eat iron-rich foods if there's considerable blood loss, including pumpkin seeds, liver, egg yolk, sunflower seeds, lentils, oats, cashews, buckwheat, and supplements such as blackstrap molasses, wheat germ, and brewer's yeast.

✓ Take sitz baths daily, if possible, to improve circulation and reduce fibroid size.

✓ Remember that surgically removed fibroids usually return.

✓ Remember, also, that fibroids shrink or even disappear during menopause unless you take estrogen.

✓ Eat three to four servings of whole grain cereals or breads daily to benefit from their antiestrogenic lignins.

✓ Ingest lignins in other foods: barley, corn, brown rice and whole wheat.

✓ Eat more fresh, green vegetables and protein-rich foods such as chicken, fish, and tofu.

✓ Drink herbal teas instead of coffee.

✓ Get a second opinion if your doctor recommends a hysterectomy, inasmuch as there are now other options for disabling fibroids: burning or freezing them or a procedure called embolization: cutting off their blood supply and starving them.

And Try This!

If bleeding is excessive, raspberry leaf tea—a cup three times daily—is helpful in restoring lost vitamins A, B, C, and E and the minerals calcium, iron, and phosphorus.

Did You Know?

Four protective factors against developing fibroids have been discovered in small studies: (1) having delivered two live children, (2) being normal in weight, (3) being athletic, and (4) eating liberal amounts of fruits, vegetables, and fish.

Varicose Veins

Added evidence in the "life is not fair" department is the statistic that women are four times more likely to develop varicose veins (enlarged and elongated veins) than men. And worse yet is the honest fact that they cannot be reversed. But there is some good news—they can be prevented and improved, sometimes dramatically, by natural methods.

Recognizing Varicose Veins

- Veins (usually in the legs) can appear thick, cordlike, bluish in color or spidery
- Sore legs and/or cramps
- Heavy feeling in the legs
- Swelling
- Itching

What Are the Causes of Varicose Veins?

In varicose situations, tiny valves in the veins are not strong enough to close completely, so blood backs up, collects, and bulges in the veins. Contributing factors can include:

- Family history
- Straining in bowel movements
- Heavy lifting
- Stress of pregnancy
- Obesity
- Lack of exercise
- Long hours of standing or sitting in one place
- Tight-fitting clothes
- Nutritional deficiencies (especially vitamin C)
- Heart disease
- Smoking

What You Can Take

Nutrients

Name	Dosage	Benefits
Vitamin A	10,000 IU daily	Promotes healing, especially when taken with zinc.
Vitamin B-complex	100 mg daily	Helpful against varicose veins.
Vitamin C	500 mg three times daily	Strengthens capillaries and improves circulation.
Vitamin E	400 IU daily	Improves circulation.
Flavonoids	1,000 mg of rutin or hesperidin daily	Works with vitamin C to strengthen capillaries and improve circulation.
Zinc	15–30 mg daily	Promotes healing, especially when taken with vitamin A.

Herbs

Name	Dosage	Benefits
Bromelain	500 mg three times daily	An enzyme derived from pineapple that is useful in improving the function and appearance of varicose veins.
Butcher's broom	100 mg after each meal	Helpful in dealing with inflammatory varicose conditions.
Gotu kola	Extract of 120 mg daily	Enhances blood flow through areas of varicose veins, and works with vitamin C to strengthen collagen and the structural integrity of veins.

Name	Dosage	Benefits
Horse chestnut	500 mg root bark capsules three times daily	Discourages inflammation, water retention, and capillary fragility.

What You Can Do

✓ Avoid straining for bowel movements (*see* CONSTIPATION).
✓ Avoid tight-fitting clothes such as girdles and garters.
✓ Avoid low-fiber, highly processed foods.
✓ Avoid sugar and other refined carbohydrates.
✓ Avoid alcohol.
✓ Don't smoke.
✓ Don't lift objects beyond your strength.
✓ Maintain a healthy body weight (*see* OVERWEIGHT).
✓ Exercise regularly.
✓ Drink at least 8–10 glasses of pure spring water daily.
✓ When standing for long periods of time, try to take as frequent breaks as possible and walk for 5–10 minutes.
✓ Eat a piece of fresh fruit or a vegetable with each meal.
✓ Eat foods high in vitamin A, including eggs, milk, cheese, cream, butter, yogurt, salmon, bass, halibut, mackerel, herring, whitefish, sardines, tuna, clams, shrimp, beef, chicken, pistachios, pecans, walnuts, lentils, and soybeans.
✓ Eat foods high in vitamin C, including rose hips, acerola cherries, guavas, black currants, red peppers, oranges, grapefruit and other citrus fruits, cabbage, papayas, cantaloupe, and tomatoes.
✓ Eat foods high in vitamin E, including sunflower seeds, whole wheat, peanuts, cashews, almonds, walnuts, corn oil, soy oil, soy lecithin, spinach, asparagus, broccoli, oats, and avocados.
✓ Eat foods high in zinc, including seafood, sardines, oysters, soybeans, soy lecithin, kelp, legumes, meat, liver, eggs, brewer's yeast, mushrooms, poultry, whole grains, and pumpkin and sunflower seeds.

And Try This!

Try wearing elastic support stockings for varicose veins of the lower leg to help prevent swelling.

Did You Know?

Varicose veins occur most often in the calves and the inside of the thigh. However, they are not restricted to the legs. Hemorrhoids, for example, are a form of varicose veins of the rectum or anus.

Vitiligo (White Spots or Patches)

I call vitiligo (white spots or patches on the skin) a minor-major ailment because it's a condition that few researchers study since it doesn't present life-or-death consequences. This is sad for two reasons. The first is that these abnormal skin colorations are often embarrassing and cause emotional stress. The second is that it almost always indicates a person is undernourished, something that can lead to more serious problems.

Recognizing Vitiligo

- Painless white spots or patches on the skin
- Spots tend to develop on both sides of the body in similar locations
- Spots may vary in number or size, and are surrounded by dark borders

What Are the Causes of Vitiligo?

Vitiligo is brought about by the destruction of melanocytes, cells that produce melanin pigment that create normal skin color. Contributing factors are believed to include:

- Family history
- Poor digestion (lack of hydrochloric acid in the stomach)
- Lack of para-aminobenzoic acid (PABA)
- Injury to the skin
- Weak immune system

What You Can Take

Nutrients

Name	Dosage	Benefits
Vitamin B-complex	100 mg daily	Necessary for maintaining the biochemical balance of all B vitamins when supplementing with any single B vitamin individually.
Vitamin B$_{12}$	1,000 mcg injections every two weeks	Folic acid can hide symptoms of vitamin B$_{12}$ deficiency. Thus vitamin B$_{12}$ should be supplemented with folic acid.
Vitamin C	1,000 mg daily	Proven useful against vitiligo.
Folic acid	1–10 mg daily	Proven useful against vitiligo.
Hydrochloric acid	Formula consisting of 648 mg of betaine hydrochloride and 130 mg of pepsin	Helpful if there are digestive problems.
Para-aminobenzoic acid (PABA)	200 mg daily	Deficiencies linked to vitiligo.

Herbs

Name	Dosage	Benefits
Khellin extract	120–160 mg daily	Only known herb shown to be effective for treating vitiligo.

What You Can Do

✓ Protect vitiligo spots from the sun either by wearing protective clothing or using strong sunscreen.
✓ Eat foods high in vitamin B$_{12}$, including liver, sardines, mackerel, herring, red snapper, flounder, salmon, lamb, Swiss cheese, blue cheese, eggs, haddock, beef, halibut, anchovies, chicken, turkey, milk, and butter.
✓ Eat foods high in folic acid, including whole grains, wheat germ, bran, brown rice, liver, milk, beef, barley, chicken,

tuna, salmon, lentils, legumes, brewer's yeast, cheese, oranges, mushrooms, and green leafy vegetables.

✓ Eat foods high in vitamin C, including rose hips, acerola cherries, guavas, black currants, red peppers, oranges, grapefruit and other citrus fruits, cabbage, papayas, cantaloupe, and tomatoes.

And Try This!

Try applying walnut juice to affected areas. While this is not a cure for vitiligo, it works as a cosmetic cover-up until the condition can be reversed by other means.

Did You Know?

One of the most significant reports on vitiligo was published many decades ago in the *Nebraska State Medical Journal*. Dr. H. W. Francis had an acute case of vitiligo himself, and finding that the parietal cells in his stomach were not producing enough hydrochloric acid, he took 15 cubic centimeters before each meal for 2 years. His vitiligo disappeared. Put on this regimen, three of his vitiligo patients had the same results. His conclusion? Improper digestion of food causes a loss of essential nutrients needed to maintain consistent skin color.

Warts

Before she had spoken a word to me, the new patient, a lovely young woman, burst into tears. As the tears ran down her cheeks, she raised her hands, the backs toward me, and they were covered with horny raised warts of all sizes. It was always embarrassing for others to see them. However, it was much more so when on a romantic evening her date reached over to hold her hand, and she abruptly pulled it away, fearing he would think she had some horrible disease. "I've had them burned off, but sooner or later, they come back," she explained with such dismay you would have thought we were discussing a terminal illness rather than a harmless, if unattractive, case of common warts.

Recognizing Warts

Warts are irregular growths on the skin most often found on the hands, fingers, feet, face and scalp. While they may vary wildly in size and shape, they tend to be rough and round with the following additional characteristics:

- Black, brown, gray, or yellow in color
- Hard to the touch
- Can appear singly or in clusters
- Usually pain free

What Are the Causes of Warts?

Warts are caused by human papilloma viruses, of which there are more than fifty different types, most being highly contagious. While they can occur anywhere on the body, they tend to develop on the areas of skin exposed to the most wear and tear such as the hands and feet. A state of weak immunity may also increase the likelihood of contracting warts.

What You Can Take

Nutrients

Name	Dosage	Benefits
Vitamin A	50,000 IU daily for two weeks *Warning:* Pregnant or pregnancy-eligible women should take no more than 10,000 IU daily.	A good start for enhancing the immune system before applying topical treatments.
Vitamin C	1,000 mg three times daily	A good start for enhancing the immune system before applying topical treatments.
Vitamin E	400 IU daily	A good start for enhancing the immune system before applying topical treatments.

What You Can Do

✓ Treat warts on the inside as well as the outside, and be patient for results.

✓ Prepare for topical applications as follows: Wash wart-covered hands and soak them in a basin of warm water for 10–15 minutes to get rid of soap residue and open pores.

✓ Apply contents of a 400 IU vitamin E capsule to warts before bedtime and cover them loosely with a Band-Aid.

✓ Use other alternate topicals, including aloe vera, a paste made from crushing a 100 or 250 mg vitamin C tablet and adding water, garlic oil, tea tree oil, goldenseal tincture, or the milky substance that comes from breaking dandelion stems.

✓ Eat foods high in vitamin A, including eggs, milk, cheese, cream, butter, yogurt, salmon, bass, halibut, mackerel, herring, whitefish, sardines, tuna, clams, shrimp, beef, chicken, pistachios, pecans, walnuts, lentils, and soybeans.

✓ Eat foods high in vitamin C, including rose hips, acerola cherries, guavas, black currants, red peppers, oranges, grapefruit and other citrus fruits, cabbage, papayas, cantaloupe, and tomatoes.

✓ Eat foods high in vitamin E, including sunflower seeds, whole wheat, peanuts, cashews, almonds, walnuts, corn oil, soy oil, soy lecithin, spinach, asparagus, broccoli, oats, and avocados.

✓ Know that warts often simply go away on their own without causing any harm.

And Try This!

You might consider the Gypsy remedy for warts (see below): Break a dandelion stem and drip its milky white fluid on the wart several times daily. After 3–4 days, the wart should darken and fall off. The one problem with this remedy is the potential harm from insecticides that may have been sprayed on the dandelions. Therefore, try to buy dandelion juice at your health food store and apply it.

Did You Know?

History tells us that at the turn of the twentieth century Gypsy wagons that traveled the country would stop near a lawn full of dandelions and occupants would swarm over the yard, quickly cutting and gathering dandelion stems. The juice from the stems was used not only for warts but for various skin lesions as well. The Gypsies also made dandelion wine from it. However, drinking this intoxicant did nothing for their warts.

Wrinkles

"Little dabs of powder, little dabs of paint, make a girl's complexion look like what it ain't." What this schoolkid's rhyme lacks in good English, it makes up in good sense, because one of the first things a girl in puberty learns is to powder over her skin blemishes. One of the last things she learns is how to prevent blemishes from happening. It's the same with people whose skin ages way before its time. As the years pass and wrinkles appear, makeup can't make up for all the abuses the skin has suffered from exterior and interior forces. By recognizing these forces and knowing how to deal with them, you can prevent or at least delay the appearance of wrinkles and reduce them once they are a reality.

Recognizing Wrinkles

Tiny lines (crow's feet) around the eyes tend to be the first sign of wrinkles. Lines and cracks around the lips (monkey lines) and cheeks are also typical early indicators of more trouble to come.

What Are the Causes of Wrinkles?

Wrinkles are caused by a lack of elasticity in the skin. Contributing factors may include the following:

- Sun exposure
- Arid desert climate
- Aging
- Smoking and secondhand smoke
- Environmental pollution
- Automobile exhaust
- Stress
- Lack of exercise

- Fluoride (mainly from fluoridated water)
- Nutritional deficiencies (especially vitamin C and vitamin B_2)
- Repetitive facial motions such as squinting or frowning
- Overuse of cosmetics that dry out the skin

What You Can Take

Nutrients

Name	Dosage	Benefits
Vitamin A	10,000 IU daily	Protects mucus membranes of the skin and helps reverse wrinkles.
Vitamin B-complex	100 mg daily	Contains vitamin B_2, which blocks the formation of monkey lines (vertical wrinkles or cracks between the nose and upper lip).
Vitamin C	500 mg three times daily	Critical to making collagen.
Vitamin E	800 IU daily	Helps compensate for stress and the wrinkles it causes.
Evening primrose oil	Two 500 mg capsules three times daily	Contains linoleic acid, which promotes healthy skin.
Magnesium	500 mg daily	Prevents calcium from migrating to collagen, which can create wrinkles.
Silica	15–25 mg daily in vegetal silica extracted from the herb horsetail	Promotes collagen production and skin elasticity.
Shark liver oil, which contains squalene	570 mg softgel twice daily	Helps moisturize skin.

What You Can Do

- ✓ Avoid excessive sun exposure.
- ✓ Avoid drinking fluoridated water and products you know contain fluoride.
- ✓ Drink at least 8–10 glasses of pure spring water daily.
- ✓ Don't smoke and avoid secondhand smoke.
- ✓ Avoid alcohol and caffeine.
- ✓ Minimize your use of cosmetics.
- ✓ Work to relieve stress (*see* STRESS).
- ✓ Exercise regularly.
- ✓ Take saunas that promote the sweating out of toxins that cause wrinkles.
- ✓ Apply vitamin C and/or vitamin E cream to wrinkles.
- ✓ Apply moisturizing creams containing hyaluronic acid or squalene.
- ✓ Keep a humidifier going to make household air moist.
- ✓ Place plants in all rooms to supply more oxygen to the air.
- ✓ Eat foods high in iron, including brewer's yeast, soy lecithin, pumpkin and sesame seeds, wheat germ, blackstrap molasses, liver, eggs, millet, lentils, walnuts, almonds, raisins, and oats.
- ✓ Eat foods high in vitamin C, including rose hips, acerola cherries, guavas, black currants, red peppers, oranges, grapefruit and other citrus fruits, cabbage, papayas, cantaloupe, and tomatoes.
- ✓ Eat foods high in copper, including mushrooms, liver, wheat germ, blackstrap molasses, hazelnuts, Brazil nuts, walnuts, cashews, salmon, ginseng, lentils, barley, and bananas.
- ✓ Eat foods high in magnesium, including blackstrap molasses, sunflower seeds, wheat germ, almonds, hazelnuts, Brazil nuts, pecans, walnuts, soybeans, soy lecithin, oats, barley, salmon, corn, avocados, bananas, cheese, tuna, and potatoes.
- ✓ Eat foods high in vitamin E, including sunflower seeds, whole wheat, peanuts, cashews, almonds, walnuts, corn oil, soy oil, soy lecithin, spinach, asparagus, broccoli, oats, and avocados.
- ✓ Eat foods high in vitamin A, including eggs, milk, cheese, cream, butter, yogurt, salmon, bass, halibut, mackerel, her-

ring, whitefish, sardines, tuna, clams, shrimp, beef, chicken, pistachios, pecans, walnuts, lentils, and soybeans.

✓ Eat foods high in vitamin B_2, including brewer's yeast, liver, royal jelly, bee pollen, almonds, wheat germ, eggs, cheese, millet, chicken, mushrooms, soybeans, sunflower seeds, lamb, peas, blackstrap molasses, cottage cheese, sesame seeds, lentils, whole rye, turkey, and broccoli.

And Try This!

Try the Japanese health custom of brushing your body for 10 minutes daily with a loofah sponge brush. It promotes better blood circulation in the skin and is an effective means of removing dead cells.

Did You Know?

Cherokee Indians brushed their skin with dried corncobs to make it more attractive and healthy. For the same reasons, Comanche Indians brushed their skin with Texas river bottom sand—an example copied by Texas rangers in the late nineteenth century.

Resource Section

Companies

The following companies have a number of products listed in this resource section. Companies with only one product listed have their toll-free numbers and websites listed along with their products.

Carlson® Laboratories
800-323-4141
www.carlsonlabs.com

Carotec, Inc.
1-800-522-4279

Healthy Origins®
1-888-228-6650

Jarrow Formulas™
1-800-726-0886
www.jarrow.com

MegaFood
800-848-2542
www.megafood.com

N.E.E.D.S.
1-800-634-1380
www.needs.com

Omega Nutrition
1-800-661-3529
www.omeganutrition.com

Source Naturals®
800-815-2333
www.sourcenaturals.com

Swedish Herbal Institute
1-800-774-9444
www.adaptogen.com

Tishcon Corporation
1-800-848-8442
www.tishcon.com

Tree of Life®
www.treeoflife.com

Tyler, Inc.
1-800-869-9705
www.tyler-inc.com

Important Products Not Previously Mentioned In This Book

Tahiti Traders
1-800-842-5309   *www.tahititraders.com*

Tahiti Trader's Noni Juice
The noni plant contains naturally occurring vitamins, minerals, enzymes, beneficial alkaloids, co-factors, plant sterols, antioxidants,

phytonutrients, and bioflavonoids. It has been used for a wide variety of health problems, including pain relief, sinus infections, arthritis, digestive disorders, colds and flu, headaches (including migraines), infections, menstrual problems, injuries, skin disorders, heart disease, type II diabetes, and more. Tahiti Trader's noni juice has an extremely high concentration of noni fruit per ounce. This is a terrific noni product.

Proper Nutrition, Inc.
1-800-555-8868   *www.propernutrition.com*

Intestive™

This all-natural dietary supplement offers total gastrointestinal support to sufferers of IBS (Irritable Bowel Syndrome) and those with general intestinal and bowel complaints. Reports and recent research by Proper Nutrition indicate that Intestive is effective in reducing symptoms related to IBS, including diarrhea and constipation, and in correcting leaky gut. The predominant ingredient in Intestive is Seacure®, a whole food concentrate from white fish that provides high quality protein in the form of bioactive peptides and biogenic amines, omega-3 fatty acids, and minerals, phospholipids, and other valuable nutrients present in fish. Dietary peptides are protein fractions that have action in the body beyond their nutritive value as a protein. The process used to produce Seacure was developed 40 years ago in an effort to transform underutilized fish into a supplement to combat world malnutrition. Clinical trials and use by health care practitioners later identified Seacure's effectiveness in intestinal healing and a history of safety, with no known side effects. Seacure is now available for the first time directly to the consumer in Intestive, enhanced with the added benefits of colostrum, free of lactose and casein, and boswellia, and anti-inflammatory herb. Intestive is available in capsule form.

SUNLEAF LABS
1-888-640-8280

Sunleaf Cellulite Reduction System
1. SUNLEAF CELLULITE REDUCTION CREAM

    A synergistic alliance of ingredients such as the herb centella asiatica, which, in combination with other herbs like siegesbeckia, camellia senensis, horsetail and others, has proven, in scientific studies, to reduce or eliminate the lumpy bulges we call cellulite, and repair damaged collagen support fibers.

Other natural ingredients, such as essential oils, MSM, noni extract, and alpha hydroxy acid, lend a support to the formula.

2. SUNLEAF DERMAL ANTIOX FORMULA
An encapsulated blend of ten potent antioxidants, which strengthen, repair, and protect the skin from the inside. This formula works on the cellular level.

Sunleaf Stretch Mark Repair System

1. SUNLEAF STRETCH MARK REPAIR CREAM
The natural transdermal delivery system enables the herb horsetail (which has a high concentration of silica) along with collagen, elastin, essential oils and other natural ingredients, to suffuse the tissues with their potent regenerative properties in order to repair or prevent stretch marks.

2. SUNLEAF DERMAL ANTIOX FORMULA
An encapsulated blend of ten potent antioxidants, which strengthen, repair, and protect the skin from the inside. This formula works on the cellular level.

Sunleaf Varicose Vein/Spider Vein Reduction System

1. SUNLEAF VEIN AND CAPILLARY FORMULA
A scientific blend of herbs, vitamins, enzymes and antioxidants, which have been shown in controlled clinical studies to reduce inflammation and pressure in blood vessels, repair weakened vessel walls, and improve circulation, visibly reducing the size and turgidity of distended veins and capillaries.

2. SUNLEAF SPIDER VEIN REPAIR CREAM
Contains vitamins C, E, and K, along with essential oils and a very effective transdermal delivery system, which enables the potent healing agents to penetrate to the cellular level.

3. SUNLEAF DERMAL ANTIOX
An encapsulated blend of ten potent antioxidants. This formula supports the other two formulas in the system through the proven action of its ingredients: strengthening and repair of damaged tissues, reduction of inflammation, and cellular protection.

Supplements

Listed here are nutritional supplements that are featured in this book. We have endeavored to find the best companies that carry these supplements. If you cannot find a particular product, contact your local health food store for assistance.

Acidophilus (Probiotics)

Probiotics use acidophilus and other strains of beneficial microflora to promote colon health. They are available from the following companies:

MegaFood

MegaFlora™

Broad spectrum probiotic complex containing 14 strains of noncompeting beneficial microflora. MegaFlora's synergistic strains produce many health promoting factors, which include: pH balancing and bacteriocin to discourage pathogenic bacteria; immune system support; volatile fatty acids that support the mucosal shield of the intestinal tract and the vagina; short chain fatty acids that control pathogenic bacteria and maintain mucus membrane integrity; natural beneficial acids such as lactic acid, acetic acid and formic acid; and free radical scavengers. Each easy-to-digest vegicap delivers 20 billion viable cells in a non-dairy base.

Source Naturals®

Life Flora™

Acidophilus/Bifidus Complex. Each 300 mg capsule contains 3 billion viable cells of freeze-dried bifidus and DDS-1 acidophilus.

Each 500 mg capsule contains 5 billion viable cells of freeze-dried bifidus and DDS-1 acidophilus. Also available in powder form.

Alpha Lipoic Acid

Available from the following companies:

Carlson® Laboratories

Alpha Lipoic Acid

Available in 100mg and 300mg tablets.

Carotec

Alpha Lipoic Acid

Each capsule contains 150mg of alpha lipoic acid.

Jarrow Formulas™

Alpha Lipoic Sustain 300

Each tablet contains 300 mg of alpha lipoic acid in a sustained release format to minimize gastric irritations and blood sugar fluctuations.

Source Naturals®

Alpha Lipoic Acid

For immune system support. Stimulates glutathione production. Available in 50 mg, 100 mg, and 200 mg tablets.

Andrographis Paniculata

Swedish Herbal Institute
Kan Jang®

Scandinavia's best-selling cold and flu tablet.

Each tablet contains 300mg of standardized andrographis paniculata (root) extract. Available in health food stores.

Antioxidants

Available from the following companies:

Carlson®
Aces Gold®

Contains vitamins A, C, E, selenium, and 12 more active nutrients or antioxidants, including CoQ10. Available in softgels.

MegaFood
Antioxidant DailyFoods® Vitamin, Mineral & Herbal Formula

Contains vitamins A, C and E, zinc and selenium. DailyFoods® FoodState® nutrients are 100% Whole Food and can be taken at any time throughout the day, even on an empty stomach. Available in tablet form.

Source Naturals®
Tocotrienol Antioxidant Complex™

Each softgel contains a total of 34 mg of tocotrienols (29.8 mg gamma-tocotrienol, 3 mg alpha-tocotrienol, and 1.3 mg delta-tocotrienol) and 100 IU of vitamin E (d-alpha tocopherol).

Swedish Herbal Institute
Chisandra Adaptogen®

One of the most powerful antioxidants known to science. Each tablet contains 100 mg of standardized schizandra chinensis (fruit) extract and 100 mg of standardized acanthopanax senticosus (root) extract.

Tishcon Corporation (raw goods supplier)
Super Antioxidant Supreme

Two softgels contain 200 IU of vitamin E (d-alpha-tocopherol plus mixed tocopherols), vitamin B-6, B-12, folic acid, selenium, alpha lipoic acid, lutein, lycopene, 1-glutathione, and other powerful nutrients.

Tishcon's Super Antioxidant Supreme is available from the following companies:

Phytotherapy: 201-891-1104
Epic: 1-800-866-0978

Optimum Health: 1-800-228-1507
Doctor's Preferred: 1-800-304-1708
Solanova: 1-800-200-0456

Biotin

Carlson®
Available in 1000 mcg tablets

Bromelain

Jarrow Formulas™
Bromelain 1000
  Each tablet contains 500 mg of bromelain (2000 GDU [Gelatin Digesting Units] per g) providing 1000 GDU per tablet or 1667 MCU (Milk Clotting Units).

Source Naturals®
Bromelain
  Each tablet contains 500 mg of bromelain (2,000 GDU per g).

Calcium
Available from the following companies:

Carlson®
Chelated Cal-Mag
  Two tablets contain 400 mg calcium and 200 mg magnesium from 333mg of calcium and magnesium chelates.

Omega Nutrition
Calcium-Magnesium Liquid (from Holistic Enterprises)
  Liquid Life Essential Night Formula is a mineral-rich formula with a pleasant coconut flavor that is designed to help tissue repair and calcium assimilation while you sleep. Suitable for all members of the family.

Charcoal

Source Naturals®
Each capsule contains 260 mg of pure activated charcoal.

Chromium
Available from the following companies:

Carlson®
Chelated Chromium
(Chelated Minerals)

Each tablet contains 200 mcg of chromium provided from 9mg of chromium glycinate chelate and complex.

Carotec
Chromium Polynicotinate and Gymnema Sylvestre
Each capsule contains 150 mcg of chromum polynicotinate and 300 mg of gymnema sylvestre extract.

Source Naturals®
Ultra Chromium GTF™
Chromium Picolinate/ ChromeMate® Complex
Each tablet contains 100 mcg of ChromeMate® chromium, 100 mcg of chromium picolinate, and .9 mg of niacin.

Tree of Life
Chromium Picolinate
Available in 200 mcg and 400 mcg tablets.

Coenzyme Q10
Available from the following companies:

Carlson®
Co-Q10
Available in 10 mg, 30 mg, 50 mg, 100 mg and 200 mg softgels.

Carotec
Co-Q10
Each softgel contains 100mg co-enzyme Q-10 with 50 mg palm tocotrienols and 200 mg of virgin coconut oil as the carrier.

Source Naturals®
Coenzyme Q10
Available in 30 mg and 100 mg softgels.

Tishcon Corporation (raw goods supplier)
Hydrosoluble CoQ10 with high bioavailability. Comes in soft-sules® (softgels).
Q-Gel®: 15 mg
Q-Gel® Forte: 30 mg
Q-Gel® Plus: with 50 mg alpha lipoic acid and 100 IU natural vitamin E
Q-Gel® Ultra: 60 mg
Carni-Q-Gel®: with 30 mg CoQ10 and 250 mg L-carnitine

Tishcon's CoQ10 products are available from the following companies:

Bio Energy Nutrients (a division of Whole Foods):
1-800-627-7775
Physiologics (a division of Whole Foods): 1-800-765-6775
CountryLife: 631-231-1031
Solanova: 1-800-200-0456
Phytotherapy: 201-891-1104
Nutrimedika: 1-800-688-7462
Swanson: 1-800-437-4148
Jordets: 1-888-816-7676
Epic: 1-800-866-0978
Optimum Health: 1-800-228-1507
Doctor's Preferred: 1-800-304-1708

Omega-3 Essential Fatty Acids

Taking Omega-3 oils in supplement form is recommended for many conditions. This is because omega-3 is part of the essential fatty acids that are necessary for health. It is found in fish oils—such as cod liver and salmon—flaxseed oil, as well as in non-fish, micro-algae form (Neuromins® DHA).

DHA (essential fatty acid)

DHA, an essential fatty acid necessary for life, is available in a non-fish, micro-algae form (for those who don't want to use fish products). Look for a product called Neuromins® DHA (in softgel form). Because of the importance of this product, several leading supplement companies are marketing Neuromins® DHA to health food stores and other stores. Listed below are companies—along with their customer service numbers—who can direct you where to obtain this product in your area:

BioDynamax (AMRION):   1-800-926-7525
Natrol®:   1-800-326-1520
Nature's Way: 1-800-962-8873
Solaray (Nutraceutical Corp.):   1-800-683-9640
Solgar: 1-800-645-2246
Source Naturals: 1-800-815-2333
Your Life (Leiner):   1-800-533-8482

Neuromins® DHA is available at health food stores everywhere, including the following:

Vitamin Shoppe:	1-800-223-1216
Vitamin World:	1-800-645-1030
Whole Foods Markets:	1-800-901-0094
Wild Oats:	1-800-494-WILD

Mail-order sources for Neuromins® DHA:

| Vitamin Shoppe: | 1-800-223-1216 |
| Puritan's Pride: | 1-900-645-1030 |

On-line sources for Neuromins® DHA (Search words: "Neuromins" or "DHA"):

www.vitaminshoppe.com
www.mothernature.com
www.drugstore.com
www.puritan.com

Evening Primrose Oil

Source Naturals®

Each softgel contains 500 mg of Evening Primrose Oil, providing 50 mg of GLA (gamma-Linoleic Acid) and 350 mg of Linoleic Acid. Hexane free.

Fish Oils (high in essential fatty acids)

Available from the following companies:

Carlson® Laboratories

Norwegian Cod Liver Oil

Bottled in liquid form. High in omega-3 and other essential fatty acids and vitamin E. Available in natural and lemon-flavored. Can be mixed into food.

Norwegian Salmon Oil

Each softgel contains 1000 mg of salmon oil. Two softgels provide 710 mg of total omega-3 fatty acids, including EPA (Eicosapentaenoic Acid), DHA (Docosahexaenoic Acid), DPA (Docosapentaenoic Acid) and ALA (Alpha-Liolenic Acid).

Super-DHA™

Each softgel contains 1000 mg of a special blend of fish body oils, including menhaden and sardines, which are high in DHA (Docosahexaenoic Acid) and EPA (Eicosapentaenoic Acid). This product is unique because it supplies as much as 500 mg of DHA and 200 mg of EPA.

Super Omega-3 Fish Oils

Contains a special concentrate of fish body oils from deep, cold-water fish, including mackerel and sardines, which are especially rich in EPA and DHA. Each softgel provides 570 mg of total omega-3 fatty acids consisting of EPA (Eicosapentaenoic Acid), DHA (Docosahexaenoic Acid), and ALA (Alpha-Liolenic Acid).

Flaxseed

Omega Nutrition
Hi-Lignan Nutri-Flax Capsules

Contains 550mg powder per capsule. A high-lignan fiber product with 7.9 mg of lignans per three-capsule (1,650 mg) serving. Lignans are the metabolism-balancing phytochemicals in flax. Flaxseed fiber contains 30% more ligans than whole flax seed.

Flaxseed Oil
Available from the following companies:

Matol
Omega 3-6-9

A rich source of omega 3, omega 6 and omega 9 essential fatty acids. Made from organic flaxseed—a major source of omega 3—enriched with GLA (gamma linolenic acid), high in dietary lignans and carotenoids. Available in liquid form.

Tree of Life®
High Lignan Flax Oil

Contains all the antioxidants of their original Organic Flax Oil plus the added benefits of high fiber lignans. Bottled in liquid form. Available in health food stores.

FOS (Fructooligosaccharides)
Available from the following companies:

Source Naturals®
NutraFlora® FOS

NutraFlora is a complex of fructooligosaccharides (FOS)—a group of naturally occurring carbohydrates that are indigestible by humans but serve as "food" for friendly flora, helping to increase their numbers in the body. Available in 1,000 mg tablets and powder form.

Garlic
Available from the following companies:

Source Naturals®
Garlic Oil
  Odorless and tasteless. Each softgel contains garlic oil extracted from 500 mg of fresh garlic bulb, in a base of soybean oil.

Wakunaga of America
1-800-421-2998
www.kyolic.com
Kyolic® Aged Garlic Extract (AGE)
  The most scientifically researched garlic product in the world (over 220 studies). Available in capsules as well as in liquid form (that can be added to food).

Glucosamine

Jarrow Formulas™
Glucosamine Sulfate 500/1000
Glucosamine sulfate 2KCI, in 500 mg capsules and 1000mg Quik-Solv™ tablets. Sodium-free.

Glucosamine Mega 1000™
  Each Quik-Solv™ tablet contains 1000mg of glucosamine hydrochloride HCI. Sodium-free.

Glutathione
Available from the following companies:

Carlson® Laboratories
Glutathione Booster™
  Provides the body with the nutrients needed to elevate or maintain healthy glutathione and glutathione peroxidase levels. Each capsule contains vitamins C and E, riboflavin (vitamin B-2), selenium, n-acetyl cysteine, milk thistle extract (silymarin), garlic, alpha lipoic, L-glutamine, L-glycine, asparagus concentrate, and glutathione.

Source Naturals®
L-Glutathione
Available in 50 mg tablets.

Chem-Defense™
  Molybdenum/ glutathione complex. Helps to remove toxins from the body. Each orange-flavored tablet contains 1.6 mg of riboflavin (as 2.25 mg flavin mononucleotide [Coenzymated™]), 120 mcg of molybdenum (as molybdenum aspartate citrate) and 50 mg

of glutathione. Taken sublingually (under the tongue) for direct absorption into the bloodstream.

Tyler, Inc.
Recancostat® 400

Each capsule contains 400 mg of reduced L-glutathione along with beet root, black currant, bilberry, elderberry, L-cysteine, and other ingredients. Terrific precursor for glutathione in the body.

Grape Seed or Pine Bark Extract
Available from the following companies:

Carlson® Laboratories
Grape Seed Extract
Each tablet contains 130 mg of grape seed extract and 50 mg of citrus flavonoids.

Source Naturals®
Proanthodyn™
Grape Seed Extract

Each tablet contains 100mg of proanthodyn from grape seed extract.

Pycnogenol®
Proanthocyanidin Complex

Made from Atlantic pine bark. Available in 25 mg, 50 mg, 75 mg, and 100 mg tablets.

Green Lipped Mussel Extract

Oceana Products
500-897-7735   *www.oceanaproducts.com*
SeaRex™

An excellent joint formulation, containing Glycomarine™, a new anti-inflammatory compound derived from the New Zealand Green Lipped Mussel, now available as an effective remedy for arthritis sufferers. This proprietary compound is backed with more than 25 years of clinical research.

For information abut the Glycomarine raw material, contact:
Marine Nutriceutical Corporation
570-897-0351
www.marine-ingredients.com

Immune System Support

Moducare Sterinol™

A wonderful new immune enhancer that is now widely available. Moducare Sterinol is a patented blend of plant sterols and sterolins that possess a powerful immune system enhancement. It has been shown to increase natural killer cell activity in your body for anti-inflammation and infection. Moducare, researched by Professor Patrick Bouic, is used to normalize or balance immune function for the treatment of cancer, autoimmune disease, allergies and other immune-mediated diseases. Thousands of research studies have been published worldwide on plant sterols and sterolins, including 140 double-blind trials in humans. Available from the following companies:

Moducare Sterinol
877-297-7332   *www.moducare.com*

Natural Balance
800-833-8737   *www.naturalbalance.com*

(In Canada) Purity Life Health Products
800-265-2615

L-Carnitine

Jarrow Formulas™
L-Carnitine Tartrate (a superior stabilized form)

Each 250 mg capsule contains 1-carnitine (from 375 mg 1-carntine tartrate). Each 500 mg capsule contains 1-carnitine (from 750 mg 1-carnitine tartrate).

Liquid Carnitine 1000

One tablespoon (15ml) contains 1,000mg 1-carnitine (USP grade, elemental free base) and 10mg pantothenic acid (vitamin B-5 as d-calcium pantothenate).

L-Glutamine
Available from the following companies:

Jarrow Formulas™
L-Glutamine Powder

Each 1/4 teaspoon contains approximately 1,000 mg (1g) of 1-glutamine, produced by biological fermentation. Each scoop contains approximately 2,000 mg (2g) of 1-glutamine.

N.E.E.D.S.
L-Glutamine
Available in capsules, tablets and powder.

Liver Support

Source Naturals®
Liver Guard™
   Contains lipoic acid, silymarin and N-acetyl cysteine (NAC) to support healthy liver function. Also contains herbs for cleansing the liver as well as choline and inositol for preventing fat from depositing in the liver. Available in tablets.

Lycopene

Healthy Origins®
Lyc-O-Mato™
An enhanced lycopene product from Israel. Available in 15 mg softgel capsules.

Lyc-O-Mato™ Plus Seleno Excell™
   A very handy and effective combination for people who want to use both lycopene and selenium. Each capsule contains 15 mg of lycopene and 100 mcg of selenium.

Magnesium
Available from the following companies:

Carlson®
Chelated Magnesium
(Chelated Minerals)
   Two tablets contain 200 mg magnesium provided from magnesium glycinate chelate.

Liquid Magnesium
   Each soft gel contains 400 mg of liquid magnesium oxide.

Source Naturals®
Magnesium
   Each tablet contains 825 mg of malic acid and 152 mg of magnesium.

Ultra Mag™
High Efficiency Magnesium Complex
   Two tablets contain 400 mg of magnesium and 50 mg of vitamin B-6.

Tree of Life
Magnesium
   Available in 250 mg tablets.

Mail Order

N.E.E.D.S.
1-800-634-1380 *www.needs.com*
N.E.E.D.S. carries a full line of quality supplements from top companies, including Jarrow Formulas™.

Melatonin
Available from the following companies:

Jarrow Formulas™
Melatonin Sustain™
   Sustained release melatonin. Each tablet contains 1 mg melatonin, 2 mg vitamin B6 (Pyridoxine HCI) and 100 mg magnesium (from oxide).

Source Naturals®
Melatonin
   Available in 1 mg, 3 mg and 5 mg tablets.

Melatonin
   Sublingual. Available in 1 mg, 2.5 mg and 5 mg orange or peppermint flavored tablets that are taken sublingually (under the tongue) for direct absorption into the bloodstream.

MSM
Available from the following companies:

Carlson®
MSM Sulfur
   Each capsule contains 1,000 mg of MSM (methylsulfonylmethane), providing 334 mg of organic dietary sulfur.

Jarrow Formulas™
MSM
   Available in 750 mg and 100 mg capsules and 200 g and 454 g powder.

Natural Balance
1-800-833-8737   *www.naturalbalance.com*
MSM
   Available in tablets and powder.

Multivitamin and Mineral Formulation

MegaFood
LIFESTYLE™ DAILYFOODS® Vitamin, Mineral & Herbal Formula

This unique formulation delivers nutrients in the FoodState® for maximum utilization. Recent scientific studies have proven that nutrients function at their peak when consumed as they naturally occur in food. Because MegaFood's formulas are food, they are particularly effective. DAILYFOODS® FoodState® nutrients are 100% Whole FOOD and can be taken at any time throughout the day, even on an empty stomach. Available in tablet form.

Mushrooms
Available from the following companies:

Carlson®
Golden Mushroom

Each softgel provides 250 mg of Shitake mushroom powder *(lentinus edodes)* and 250 mg of Reishi mushroom powder *(ganoderma)*, plus 10 IU of natural source vitamin E.

Maitake Products, Inc.
1-800-747-7418   *www.maitake.com*
Maitake D-fraction® Extract

Studies in Japan and elsewhere indicate that this product may be effective against cancer. Every six drops contains a minimum of pure and active 6.6 mg of beta-glucan in a standardized extract.

N-Acetyl Cysteine
N-acetyl cysteine is an amino acid that is valuable for the production of glutathione in our bodies. Available from the following companies:

Carlson®
N·A·C

Available in 500 mg capsules and also available in powder.

Source Naturals®
N-Acetyl Cysteine

Available in 600 mg and 1,000 mg tablets.

Niacinamide
Available from the following companies:

Carlson®
Niacin-Amide

Cellulose-coated tablets for ease of swallowing. Available in 100mg or 500mg.

Source Naturals®
Niacinamide

Available in 100 mg and 1,500 mg time-released tablets.

PC SPES

An herbal combination that has been very effective in treating prostate cancer and dramatically reducing PSA levels. It also doesn't have as many side effects as with hormonal drugs. Available through the following company:

BotanicLab™
1-800-242-5555   *www.botaniclab.com*

BotanicLab™ is the primary distributor of PC SPES, which has had encouraging results in clinical trials involving prostate cancer patients at well-respected university research centers, including UCSF Medical Center, Columbia-Presbyterian Medical Center, the Cancer Institute of New Jersey, and the University of Kentucky. In addition, several *in vivo* and *in vitro* studies have been conducted at various well-known research laboratories and published in medical journals. For information about PC SPES, contact BotanicLab™ through their toll-free phone number or visit them on their website.

Potassium

Available from the following companies:

Carlson®
Potassium

Each table provides 99 mg of potassium from 595 mg of potassium gluconate.

Matol
KM®

A very potent and effective compound. Liquid extract for maximum absorption. Each serving of two tablespoons contains 562 mg of potassium and 14 herbs, which provide powerful essential minerals. Also available in capsules.

Source Naturals®
Potassium

Each tablet contains 99 mg of potassium (from 495 mg of potassium amino acid chelate).

Progesterone Cream
For PMS and menopause relief. Available from the following companies:

N.E.E.D.S.
Pro-Gest
Body Cream Specific
   A soothing topical cream which contains an extract of wild yam. A rich source of natural plant progesterone.

Omega Nutrition
Progestone 900™
   Fragrant, pleasant to use moisturizing cream that is easily absorbed into the skin and designed for women who cannot produce enough progesterone on their own. Contains both 900 mg of pharmaceutical-grade progesterone and 1,995 mg of dermasterone, a bioactive multi-species wild yam complex. Also recommended for osteoporosis protection.

Source Naturals®
Eternal Woman Progesterone Cream
   Made from soy, enhanced by Mexican wild yam and black cohosh root extract. Guaranteed to contain 500 mg of progesterone per ounce.

Quercetin
Available from the following companies:

Jarrow Formulas™
Quercetin 500™
   Bioflavonoid antioxidant available in 500 mg capsules.

Source Naturals®
Activated Quercetin™
   Nonallergenic bioflavonoid complex. Three tablets contain 1,000 mg quercetin, 600 mg vitamin C (magnesium ascorbate), 47 mg magnesium (magnesium ascorbate), and 300 mg bromelain (2,000 GDU per g).

NutraSpray™ Quercetin
   Seasonal bioflavonoid complex. Each spray contains 50 mg quercetin. Natural tangerine flavor.

Royal Jelly

Source Naturals®
Each capsule contains freeze-dried royal jelly equivalent to 500 mg of fresh royal jelly, in a base of rice powder.

Selenium

Healthy Origins®
Seleno Excell™
Used extensively in tests by Dr. Clark at the University of Arizona. Each tablet contains 200 mcg of selenium and 39.7 mg of calcium. A highly researched and effective selenium.

Shark Liver Oil

Scandinavian Laboratories
1-570-897-7735
Oceana®
Each soft gel contains 570 mg of purified whole shark liver oil, naturally combining 110 mg of squalene with 325 mg of diacylglycerol ethers (D.A.G.E.) and 125 mg of alkylglycerols. Also contains some omega-3 fatty acids.

Silicon

Jarrow Formulas™
BioSil™
Silicon is a crucial component of structural and connective tissues such as cartilage and collagen. It also regulates calcium deposition in bones. BioSil™ is a 30 ml solution of orthosilicic acid—the only form of biologically active silicon absorbed by the body—choline chloride and glycerine. Each drop contains 1mg of silicon as orthosilicic acid. BioSil™ has been clinically proven to be 150% (2.5 times) more bioavailable than horsetail or gel forms of silicon.

Soy

Carlson®
Easy Soy® Gold
Each tablet contains 325 mg of high isoflavone concentrate, providing 130 mg of soy isoflavones, including 60 mg of genistein and genistin, 58 mg of daidzein and daidzin, and 12 mg of glycitein and glycitin.

Swedish Flower Pollen

Graminex, L.L.C.
1-877-472-6469 *www.graminex.com*
Cernilton®

Long term clinical research supports the benefits of Cernilton®, which contains Cernitin™ flower pollen extract, in promoting healthy prostate function. Studies show a reduction in prostate volume, residual urine volume, and the improvement of voiding difficulties. Other symptoms of BPH and prostatitis may be reduced. Cernitin™ flower pollen extract may improve the conditions of liver function, smooth muscle function and immune system function. The chemical analysis of Cernitin™ flower pollen extract shows that it contains most of the vitamins, minerals, amino acids and enzymes the body needs in micro nutrient quantities. It is a standardized, virtually allergen-free whole extract of selected pollen. Four tablets contain 250 mg of pollen extract.

Turmeric

Source Naturals®
Turmeric Extract

Each tablet contains 350 mg of turmeric extract, yielding 95% curcumin, and 50 mg bromelain.

Vitamin A
Available from the following companies:

Jarrow Formulas™
Marine Beta Carotene

Beta carotene is pro-vitamin A and is converted upon absorption (at the intestines) into vitamin A only if needed. Otherwise, beta carotene functions as a singlet oxygen quencher and antioxidant. Each softgel contains 15mg of beta carotene (from the sea algae Dunaliella salina), which is equivalent to 25,000 IU of pro-vitamin A activity, as well as 5 IU of vitamin E. Available through N.E.E.D.S.

Source Naturals®
Vitamin A Palminate

Each tablet contains 10,000 IU of vitamin A (palminate).

Active A™

Each tablet contains 15,000 IU of vitamin A (beta carotene) and 10,000 IU of Vitamin A (palminate), yielding 25,000 IU of total vitamin A activity.

Tree of Life®
Vitamin A
　Each softgel contains 8,000 IU of vitamin A, from fish liver oil.

Beta Carotene
　Beta carotene is a nutrient that the body can convert to vitamin A as needed. Each softgel contains 25,000 IU of vitamin A, from carrot oil.

Vitamin A Tip
You will notice that vitamin A is recommended for many of the conditions in this book. In Germany, physicians recommend vitamin A for the prevention and treatment of many diseases. It is particularly effective when used in combination with zinc.

Vitamins A and D

Carlson®
Vitamins A and D_3
　Each softgel contains 10,000 IU of natural source vitamin A and 400 IU of natural source vitamin D_3 from fish liver oil.

Vitamin B-6

Source Naturals®
Vitamin B-6 (Pyridoxine HCL) in 50 mg, 100 mg, and 500 mg time-released tablets.

Vitamin B-12

Source Naturals®
　Each sublingual tablet contains 2,000 mcg of Vitamin B-12 (cyanocobalamin), sweetened wtih sorbitol and mannitol and flavored with natural lemon.

Vitamin B Complex
Available from the following companies:

Carlson®
B-Compleet™
　Provides all the B-vitamins plus vitamin C in a balanced formulation. Available in tablets.

Carotec
Bio B-Complex

Each capsule contains 25 milligrams of each of the "macro" B-vitamins (B-1, B-2, B-3, B-6) plus pantothenic acid; 25 micrograms of B-12 and D-biotin; 200 micrograms of folic acid; 80 mg of choline; 50 mg of inositol; 2 mg of PABA; plus 5 mg of Bioperine®, an ingredient that makes the B-vitamins and other nutrients better absorbed and metabolized.

Source Naturals®
Coenzymate™ B Complex

Contains coenzymes along with a full range of B-vitamins and CoQ10. Available in orange or peppermint flavored tablets that are taken sublingually (under the tongue) for direct absorption into the bloodstream.

Vitamin C
Available from the following companies:

Carlson®
Mild-C Chewable

Buffered form of chewable vitamin C that is non-acidic and gentle to the teeth. Each orange and tangerine flavored tablet supplies 250 mg of vitamin C and 28 mg of calcium.

MegaFood
Complex C

Vitamin C as found in food, is a very complex nutrient of which ascorbic acid is only one factor. Complex C DAILYFOODS® contains all the food factors, such as bioflavonoids, that occur in food and enhance its effectiveness. DAILYFOODS® FoodState® nutrients are 100% Whole FOOD and can be taken at any time throughout the day, even on an empty stomach. Available in 250 mg tablets.

Source Naturals®
C-500

Each tablet provides 500 mg of vitamin C (ascorbic acid) and 50 mg of rose hips.

Wellness C-1000™

Each tablet contains 1,000 mg of vitamin C and several sources of bioflavonoids and alpha-lipoic acid.

Vitamin D

Available from the following companies:

Moss Nutrition

1-800-851-5444

Bio-D-Mulsion

An oil in water emulsion in which vitamin D has been dispersed. Each drop supplies 400 IU of emulsified vitamin D. If you wish to have your dentist or physician inquire about this product, they can call Moss Nutrition.

Carlson®

Vitamin D_3

Natural source vitamin D_3 from fish liver oil. Available in 400 IU and 1,000 IU softgels.

Vitamin E

Available from the following companies:

Carotec

Vitamin E

Each softgel contains 200 IU alpha tocopherol, 75 mg gamma tocopherol, 28 mg delta tocopherol, and 1 mg beta tocopherol.

Carlson®

d-Alpha Gems™

Each tiny softgel contains 400 IU of vitamin E (d-alpha tocopherol acetate).

E-Gems® Plus

Each soft gel contains vitamin E derived from soybean oil, supplying alpha-tocopherol plus mixed tocopherols. Available in three strengths: 200 IU, 400 IU and 800 IU.

Jarrow Formulas

Oil E

Vitamin E as 100% natural form d-alpha tocopherol with mixed tocopherols. Available in 400 IU and 600 IU soft gels.

MegaFood

E & Selenium DAILYFOODS®

In foods, vitamin E and selenium are always found together. Vitamin E doesn't work without the presence of selenium and vice versa. This combination offers these two important nutrients as they naturally occur in food, and therefore provides maximum protection. DAILYFOODS® FoodState® nutrients are 100% Whole

FOOD and can be taken at any time throughout the day, even on an empty stomach. Each tablet contains 100 IU of vitamin E and 100 mg of selenium.

Source Naturals®
Vitamin E

Each softgel contains 400 IU of natural vitamin E (d-alpha-tocopherol) and 67 mg of mixed tocopherols (d-beta, d-gamma, and d-delta). In a base of soybean oil.

Tocotrienol Antioxidant Complex™

Each softgel contains a total of 34 mg of tocotrienols (29.8 mg gamma-tocotrienol, 3 mg alpha-tocotrienol, and 1.3 mg delta-tocotrienol) and 100 IU of vitamin E (d-alpha tocopherol).

Vitamins—Kosher

Freeda® Vitamins
1-800-777-3737

For those who adhere to a Kosher regimen, Freeda has been making and distributing a full line of absolutely Kosher vitamins and supplements since 1928. Call their toll-free number for information and a list of stores who carry their line.

Weight Loss Formulations

Galaxy Worldwide
1-866-USA-SLIM / 1-866-872-7546
BeSlimmer A.M. Formula

Each capsule contains chromium, ma huang, kola nut, ginger root, white willow bark, gingko biloba, bladderwrack, fo-ti, hawthorn, saw palmetto, beet (root), and boron chelate.

BeSlimmer P.M. Formula Nite Complex

Each caplet contains vitamin C, vitamin B-6, calcium, chromium, chloride, potassium, L-arginine, L-ornithine, L-lysine, valerian, glycine, GABA, L-tyrosine, L-carnitine, and melatonin.

BeSlimmer CarboBlock

Each capsule contains vitamin C, chromium, phaseolus vulgaris bean, gymnema sylvestre, garcinia cambogia, royal jelly, Siberian ginseng, American ginseng root, and vanadyl sulfate.

Zinc
Available from the following companies:

Carlson® Laboratories
Zinc
Contains zinc from zinc gluconate in 15 mg and 50 mg tablets.

Jarrow Formulas™
Zinc Balance 15™

A synergistic combination of OptiZinc™ brand zinc monomethionate and copper gluconate in a 15:1 zinc/copper ratio. Each capsule contains 15 mg of zinc (as monomethionine) and 1 mg of copper (as gluconate).

Source Naturals®
OptiZinc®

Each tablet contains 30 mg of zinc (from 150 mg of OptiZinc® zinc monomethionine)

Herbs

Astragalus Extract
Available from the following companies:

Matol
1-800-363-1890
www.matol.com
Biomune OSF™ Plus

A very effective formulation in boosting and enhancing immune function. Each capsule contains 200 mg of astragalus (root) and other ingredients, including 100 mg of dairy colostrum and whey extract (Ai/E^{10}™).

Planetary Formulas®
800-815-2333
www.sourcenaturals.com
Full Spectrum™ Astragalus Extract

Each two tablet serving combines 500 mg of standardized astragalus root extract with 500 mg of whole high grade astragalus root.

Black Elderberry Extract

Carotec
A traditional extract in syrup form to support the throat and immunity. Each bottle contains four ounces of black elderberry extract in tupelo honey.

Germanium

Jarrow Formulas™
GE-132
Pure organic germanium in 30 mg, 100 mg, and 150 mg capsules and 5 g powder.

Ginger
Available from the following companies:

Jarrow Formulas™
Freeze-Dried Ginger
  Each capsule contains 500 mg of freeze-dried ginger.

Garlic+Ginger
  Each capsule contains 500 mg of Jarro-Gar™ odor modified garlic and 200 mg of freeze-dried ginger (6:1 extract).

Gingko Biloba
Available from the following companies:

Carlson®
Gingko Biloba Plus
  Each softgel contains 40 mg of gingko biloba and 200 mg of 1-glutamine.

Jarrow Formulas™
Gingko Biloba 50:1 Liquid
  Each 1 ml contains 60 mg water soluble gingko biloba 50:1 liquid extract.

Gingko 50:1 = Grape OPC
  Each capsule contains 60 mg of gingko biloba leaf 50:1 standardized extract and 50 mg of grape seed 100:1.

Green Tea Extract

Source Naturals®
  Each tablet contains 100 mg of standardized, patented Polyphenon 60™ green tea extract, providing at least 65 mg of polyphenols.

Kava Kava

Source Naturals®
Kava-77™
  For relaxation. Each softgel contains 140 mg of kava kava root

extract *(piper methysticum)* standardized to 55% kavalactones, yielding 75 mg of kavalactones.

Olive Leaf Extract

Source Naturals®
Wellness Olive Leaf™
Each tablet contains 500 mg of olive leaf standardized extract, yielding 75 mg of oleuropein.

Pygeum Africanum

Carotec
Prostate Support Formula
Each capsule contains 100 mg of Pygeum Africanum and 200 mg of Stinging Nettle (Urtica dioca).

Herbs (tinctures extracted with alcohol)

The primary forms of delivery for herbs are capsules, tablets, and tinctures from herbal extracts. Most herbalists recommend tinctures because the herbs keep fresher and stronger when extracted with alcohol. Also, usually more of the active constituents of the herb are effectively extracted by alcohol rather than water. Listed below are three top companies who guarantee the strengths listed on the bottles of their products. You can rely on their products for quality, potency and safety.

BD Herbs
1-800-760-3739   *www.bdherbs.com*
All of the herbs used by BD Herbs are grown on their Demeter certified biodynamic home ranch, hand-harvested and extracted with certified organic alcohol. Interestingly, they grow their herbs in between rows of grapes, which are used for their very fine Frey Vineyards organic wines.

Angelica	Feverfew	St. John's Wort
German Chamomile	Organic Gingko Biloba	Valerian
Echinacea	Grape Seed	Yarrow

Gaia Herbs
1-800-831-7780
www.gaiaherbs.com
Founded by Ric Scalzo, Gaia uses only certified organic and eco-

logically wildcrafted herbs that are specifically selected and formulated to work synergistically within the body. This company also has a full line of herbs in capsules and liquid phyto-caps—a revolutionary new delivery system for liquid herbal extracts. All phyto-caps are vegetable-based and alcohol-free.

Angelica	Feverfew	Licorice Root
Astragalus	Garlic Oil	Milk Thistle
Bilberry	Ginger Root Extract	Nettle Leaf
Blue or Black Cohosh	Gingko Biloba	Pygeum Africanum
Burdock	Goldenseal	Sage
Butcher's Broom	Gotu Kola Extract	Shepherd's Purse
Cascara Sagrada	Green Tea Extract	Siberian Ginseng
Cat's Claw	Gymnema Sylvestre	Tea Tree Oil
Chamomile	Hawthorn	Urtica Dioica (nettle)
Chasteberry	Hawthorn Berry	Valerian Root
Chlorophyll	Horehound	White Willow Extract
Dandelion Root	Horse Chestnut	Yarrow Extract
Echinacea	Horsetail (a rich	Yohimbe
False Unicorn	source of silica)	Yucca
(helonias root)	Kava Kava	

Planetary Herbs/Formulas
1-800-777-5677 www.planetherbs.com

Dr. Michael Tierra, OMD, L.Ac., is one of the foremost authorities on herbal medicine in North America and has had a clinical practice for 30 years. He is the product formulator for Planetary Formulas and is an internationally recognized authority on the world's herbal traditions. Planetary Formulas carries a wide range of herbs and herbal formulas in tablets and tinctures extracted with alcohol. They also carry a line of herbs for children with glycerin added to neutralize any alcohol taste.

Herb Tip
When following this book's recommendations for herbal teas, try using tinctures from herbal extracts: to hot (almost boiling) water, add a few drops of tincture to your own taste (do not exceed the recommended dosage on the tincture bottle)

Homeopathic

Dr. Langer has found that combination (multi-ingredient) homeopathic formulas are easier to select and often more effective than single ingredient products. As a result, he uses combination formulas almost exclusively in his clinical practice. Contact Liddell Laboratories (below) for their list of combination formulas, which contain the homeopathic remedies that are recommended in this book.

Liddell Laboratories
1-800-460-7733
www.liddell.net
Liddell offers a highly effective and easy to use homeopathic line of sublingual oral sprays. These products relieve a wide range of symptoms associated with such conditions as cold and flu, sinus congestion, allergy and hay fever, back pain, sciatica, arthritis, and stress. Formulated by a physician, all of Liddell's 130 spray products contain safe and effective natural ingredients. Their new oral spray system delivers exceptional absorption by the body and these sprays have been shown to work well in combination with other products such as dietary supplements and over-the-counter or prescription drugs.

Special Resource Section (including foods, teas, juices, etc.)

Beef—Organic

Homestead Healthy Foods™
1-888-861-5670
www.homesteadhealthyfoods.com
Homestead Healthy Foods™ beef is raised in pastures on natural forages, which are certified organic and inspected annually by the certifier. Because it is raised on grass, the beef is high in omega-3 essential fatty acids. The meat is also lower in fat and free of any chemical residue, growth hormones, antibiotics or pesticides. Noted health authority, Andrew Weil, M.D., cautions people to buy organic meat and poultry because they are free of added antibiotics, which the body does not need.

Cheese—Organic
Available from the following companies:

Country Hills Organic, Inc.
330-893-2596
Pure Pastures Organic Cheese
A complete family of delicious and healthy organic cheeses that
are produced in accordance with the 1990 California Organic
Foods Act. Contry Hills' dairy farmers are overseen by the Ohio
Ecological Food and Farm Association (OEFFA) and raise their
cattle on organic grains and feed. Herds are free of chemicals, artificial growth hormones and antibiotics. All of their products are
made with 100% certified organic milk and ingredients that are
certified organic by Quality Assurance International (QAI). Their
cheeses are available in six traditional styles, including Cheddar,
Colby, Swiss and Havarti, as well as an assortment of yogurt
cheeses.

Tree of Life
Organic Cheeses, including Colby, Cheddar, Jalapeño Jack, Moz-
zarella, Provolone, and Swiss. These wonderful cheeses are available at many health food stores.

Chia Seed

The Andersen Company
760-776-1421
Chia seed was first used by the ancient Aztecs. The Andersen's
Company's chia seed is sold in one pound packages with roughly
800,000 seeds to a pound.

Flaxseeds

Omega Nutrition
Flax Of Life—Cold Milled Organic Flax Seeds
Certified-organic flax seeds, vacuum-packed in a lined, resealable
foil bag to retain freshness.

Flax Of Life—Whole Organic Flax Seeds
Certified-organic flax seeds.

Ginger Tea

Triple Leaf Tea, Inc.
1-800-552-7448   *www.tripleleaf-tea.com*
Ginger Tea
Made from 100% ginger root. Available in tea bags.

Grains

Available from the following companies:

INF—InterNatural Foods
201-909-0808
McCann's Steelcut Wholegrain Irish Oatmeal
High in B vitamins, calcium, protein and fiber, while low in fat with no added salt.

Lundberg Family Farms
530-882-4550 (ext. 319) *www.lundberg.com*
Grower and marketer of organic rice and rice products. They have an amazing variety of rices, rice cakes, etc. Reliable quality.

Green Drinks—Powdered

Available from the following companies:

Greens +®
1-800-643-1210   *www.greensplus.com*
Greens +®
   A whole living food containing concentrated sources of organic vitamins, minerals, essentials amino acids, phytochemicals, enzymes, co-enzymes, cell salts, chlorophyll, standardized herbal extracts, unique botanical extracts and soluble and insoluble plant fibers. Winner of the Peoples' Choice Award for the NNFA Market Place 2000.

Protein Greens+®
   A synergistic blend of biologically complete protein isolates and the 29 nutrient-rich superfoods found in the award-winning Greens+ ®. Available in soy protein and whey protein formulas.

Tree of Life®
Advanced Greens
   A blend of 29 nutrient-rich sea and land-based super-foods, herbs, fibrous ingredients and dairy-free probiotic cultures. Available in original and orange flavors. Naturally sweetened.

Advanced Greens with Protein
   Contains soy and whey protein. Available in lemon-lime and cinnamon spice flavors.

Wakunaga
Kyo-Greens®
   A combination of organically grown barley and wheat grasses, kelp, chlorella and brown rice. Two teaspoons provide the nutrients of a serving of deep green leafy vegetables.

Nuts, Nut Butters and Seeds—Organic
Available from the following companies:

Living Tree Community Foods
1-800-260-5534
Organically grown nuts and nut butters, including almonds (many varieties), macadamia nuts, pinenuts, pumpkin seeds, sunflower seeds, walnut quarters, raw almond butter, and raw cashew butter. They refrigerate their nuts, seeds and nut butters until the day they are shipped.

Tree of Life
Tree of Life Creamy Cashew Butter
Tree of Life Organic Sesame Tahini
Tree of Life Organic Almond Butter—Creamy or Crunchy
Organic almonds are a good source of B-vitamins, vitamin E, essential fatty acids, calcium, and other important minerals, as well as a substantial amount of protein.

Oils
Available from the following companies:

Omega Nutrition
Essential Balance Jr.
Omega's proprietary blend of five fresh-pressed oils, scientifically blended in the evolutionary 1:1 omega-3/omega-6 ratio. Contains certified organic flax, sunflower, sesame, pumpkin and borage oils. Also contains gamma-linolenic acid (GLA) and omega-6 fatty acids that diabetics often cannot produce. Formulated with a natural butterscotch flavoring that kids will love.

Flax Seed Oil
Unrefined and certified organic, grown without pesticides or artificial fertilizers and processed using Omega's exclusive omegaflo® process.

Olive Oil
Made from unrefined, extra-virgin olives that are fresh-pressed and omegaflo® bottled.

Tree of Life®
Tree of Life High Lignan Flax Oil
Contains all the antioxidants of their original Organic Flax Oil plus the added benefits of high fiber lignans. Bottled in liquid form. Available in health food stores.

Tree of Life Organic Extra Virgin Olive Oil

Bella Via Organic Extra Virgin Olive Oil
  Made from the first pressing of 100% organic olives imported from the Andalusia region of Spain.

Poultry

Sheltons Poultry, Inc.
1-800-541-1833
  Free-range chicken and turkey with no added antibiotics. Available in natural foods stores. Noted health expert, Andrew Weil, M.D., cautions people to avoid eating poultry and meat with added antibiotics, which has been linked to drug-resistant strains of disease-causing bacteria.

Seafood
Available from the following companies:

Capilano Pacific
1-877-391-WILD (9453)   *www.capilanopacific.com*
Wildfish™
  This company is a wonderful source for wild-caught salmon. Most of the salmon available in restaurants and stores are farm-raised. Usually this means medications such as antibiotics have been added to the feed, as well as synthetic coloring. Wild-caught salmon has none of these problems and a high level of omega-3 fatty acids and much less fat than farm-raised salmon. It tastes better as well. Also available: halibut, tuna and lox without any added chemicals.

New World Marketing Group
203-221-8008
Sardines
  Packed in pure virgin olive oil and virgin olive oil with garlic. Very high in omega-3 fatty acids. They also have water-packed sardines which contain less sodium. Available in natural foods stores.

Stevia

Wisdom of the Ancients®
1-800-899-9908   www.wisdomherbs.com
  Natural sweetener made from whole leaf Stevia *(Stevia rebaudiana Bertoni)* 6:1 concentrated extract. Available in concentrated tablets, liquid, and as a tea. Hundreds of scientific studies have been conducted on Stevia's effectiveness as a nutritional support for the pancreas.

Teas (Green)
Available from the following companies:

Great Eastern Sun
1-800-334-5809   www.great-eastern-sun.com

Haiku® Organic Japanese Teas

Organic Original Sencha Green Tea:
The finest grade of green leaf tea available, made from the tender young leaves of selected tea bushes, cut at the peak of their flavor, rolled, steamed, and briefly dried. Contains 100% Nagata Japanese Organic Sencha Green Tea Leaves and Buds. Available in tea bags and bulk.

Organic Original Hojicha Roasted Green Tea:
Lower in caffeine than Sencha, Hojicha has a subtle smoky and rich flavor that is quite different from that of Sencha. Contains 100% Nagata Japanese Organic Hojicha Roasted Green Tea Leaves and Stems. Available in tea bags and bulk.

Maitake Products, Inc.
1-800-747-7418   *www.maitake.com*
Mai Green™ Tea
Contains organically grown maitake mushroom and premier Japanese green tea (matcha) leaves. Low in caffeine. Available in tea bags.

The Republic of Tea
1-800-298-4TEA (4932)   *www.republicoftea.com*
Growers and marketers of certified organic teas, including green teas and herbal teas. Available in bulk or in tea bags at natural food stores, gourmet and specialty food stores, and select department stores, café and restaurants.

Triple Leaf Tea, Inc.
1-800-552-7448
Authentic traditional Chinese medicinal teas in tea bags, including different varieties of green tea. Triple Leaf has a natural method of decaffeinating green tea without using any chemical solvents. If you drink a lot of green tea and don't want caffeine, this is an ideal tea to use.

Tree of Life®
www.treeoflife.com
There are many fine healthfood stores all over the country that carry top-notch products. Many stores are supplied by an excellent

company known as Tree of Life, a distributor of high quality natural foods at moderate prices. When shopping at health food stores, you can ask for Tree of Life products. If a store doesn't carry a particular product, they can order it for you.

Tree of Life Frozen Organic Vegetables
Certified organically grown.
Broccoli
Corn
Green Peas
Spinach

Tree of Life Frozen Organic Fruit
Loaded with nutrients without any added chemicals. They are often difficult to obtain.
Strawberries
Blueberries
Raspberries

Tree of Life Frozen Smoothie Makers
Fresh-frozen chunks of 100% organic fruit. Ideal for juicing.
Banana, Rasberry, Strawberry

Tree of Life Pasta Sauce
Original and Salt-Free—in glass jars.
This organic pasta sauce is made from vine-ripened, specially selected premium tomatoes that are grown for their sweetness and flavor.

Tree of Life Organic Tamari and Shoyu
Made from organic soybeans and wheat. Excellent for steamed vegetables and fish.
Shoyu
Wheat-Free Tamari

Harmony Farms Light Soymilk
Made from certified GMO-free soybeans. Available in orange or vanilla flavors, enriched with extra vitamins and minerals.

Harmony Farm Soy Burgers
High in protein and isoflavones. Available in the following flavors: original, garlic, mushroom and onion.

Tree of Life Tofu
Third party certified organic tofu, Available in a fourteen delicious varieties, including 30% reduced fat tofu, organic baked tofu, organic oriental baked tofu, and organic island spice baked tofu.

Tree of Live Advantage\10™ Entrees

Endorsed by renowned heart pioneer, Dr. Dean Ornish. These products are all natural, vegetarian, cholesterol-free, and with less than 10% of their calories derived from fat.

Advantage\10™ Soups: Packed in single serving bowls. Cajun Black Bean, Southwestern Chili, and Tuscan Vegetable Minestrone.

Advantage\10™ Meal Entrees: Pasta Santa Fe, Mediterranean Pasta, Carribean Sweet/Sour, Vegetable Szechuan.

Advantage\10™ Pizzas: Roasted Vegetable With No Cheese, Vegetarian Pepperoni, Vegetarian Sausage/Mushroom.

Wine—Organic

Frey Vineyards

1-800-760-3739

For those who drink wine, Frey Vineyard's wines are organic and free of sulfites.

Yogurt

Brown Cow Yogurt

Yogurt is a good substitute for ice cream with only a third of the fat and a third of the calories. It is also less allergenic than milk because the lactose has been fermented. Brown Cow yogurt is pasteurized but not homogenized and therefore safer for blood vessels. It contains live active cultures and no steroids, bovine growth hormone or antibiotics. Brown Cow Yogurt is available in health food stores and many supermarkets. It is sold by Oasis Sales and Marketing. For more information on their products and where to purchase them, call Oasis at 707-824-0119.

Detoxification

When taking charge of your health, it is very important to avoid toxins in the food you eat, the water you drink, the air you breathe, and in virtually every product you use, from shampoos and toothpaste to cleansers and cosmetics. The companies listed here are of the highest quality. If you cannot find their products at your local health food store, please contact these companies directly for the store nearest you.

Dental Products

Woodstock Natural Products, Inc.
The Natural Dentist™
1-800-615-6895

Toothpaste: mint, cinnamon and fluoride-free mint
Mouth rinse: mint, cinnamon, and cherry-flavored

There is a holistic connection between the health of your teeth
and gums and your whole body. This is especially true for diabetics, who need to be vigilant about their teeth and gums because
they have a tendency to develop periodontal disease. Woodstock
Natural Products are formulated by a holistic dentist and contain
soothing and healing herbs, with no alcohol, sugar, or harsh chemicals. These products have been clinically proven to kill germs that
cause gum disease. In a study published in the *Journal of Clinical
Dentistry* in 1998, researchers at the New York University College
of Dentistry in New York City found that The Natural Dentist
toothpaste removed plaque more effectively than the leading commercial brand. The same group also found that The Natural Dentist
mouth rinse killed more germs than the leading commercial brand.

Desert Essence®
1-888-476-8647   *www.desertessence.com*
Oral Care Collection
A complete line of antiseptic and cleansing oral care products
using tea tree oil for deep cleaning and disinfecting of teeth and
gums. All products are animal and eco-friendly and made without
artificial colors, sweeteners or harsh abrasives.

Tea Tree Oil Dental Floss: creates a germ-free mouth and cleans
between teeth
Tea Tree Oil Dental Tape: provides same benefits as floss with a
wider ribbon
Tea Tree Oil Dental Pics: cleans between teeth with antiseptic
power
Tea Tree Oil Breath Freshener: contains natural and organic essential oils

Mail Order

N.E.E.D.S.
1-800-634-1380   *www.needs.com*
An excellent resource for top-notch environmental products, including the following:

Aireox Air Purifier (Model 45)
Removes mold spores, pollen dust, formaldehyde, and more.

Airoex Car Air Purifier (Model 22)
An unusual purifier for the car.

Allens Naturally
A full line of toxin-free household cleansers, including dishwashing and laundry detergents and all-purpose cleaners.

Water Filters
N.E.E.D.S. carries a variety of high-quality water filters.

Elite Shower Filter and Massager
For removing chlorine, heavy metals and bacteria.

Natural Cosmetics
Available from the following companies:

Carlson®
E-Gem® Oil Drops
Each drop contains 10 IU of vitamin E. 5000 IU of vitamin E per ½ ounce. Apply externally to aid and soften skin.

E-Gem® Organic Shampoo
Formulated with vitamin E, vitamins A and D, panthenol and protein.

Garden Fresh Soap
100% vegetarian. Contains aloe vera, avocado, cucumber, carrot oil, olive oil and other ingredients.

Jason Natural Cosmetics
1-800-JASON-05   *www.jason-natural.com*
Chamomile Liquid Satin Soap™ with Pump
Natural Sea Kelp Shampoo
   Jason Natural carries a full line of cosmetics that are free of toxic substances, including natural underarm deodorant and alcohol-free shaving cream and after-shave lotion.

Omega Nutrition
Unscented Face and Body Soap
   Made the old-fashioned way, in small batches using an early 1900's formulation. They use only food grade oils, including unrefined omegaflo® oils. Omega also carries a baby shampoo for sensitive skin and hair.

Far Infrared Therapy Sauna

High Tech Health
1-800-794-5355 *www.hightechhealth.com*

Thermal Life® Far Infrared Therapy Sauna

This highly effective low-temperature sauna (100°F to 130°F) employs heaters that emit rays at a special wavelength designed to push heavy metal toxins, including mercury and other toxins, out of the body through the sweat glands. There have been reports of high mercury levels coming down substantially—some cases have become mercury-free in 90 days. More than 300 doctors in the U.S. are now providing this therapy for their patients. The best part of this sauna is its ease of use. It requires no pre-heating, doesn't need any water, and it can be moved anywhere in the home or apartment. Unit sizes available for 1–5 persons.

Water Filter

High Tech Health, inc.
1-800-794-5355 http://*www.hightechhealth.com*
Ionizer Plus

This water filter provides superior water filtration to $\frac{1}{10}$ of a micron (below bacteria levels) and ultraviolet to eliminate viruses. The greatest benefit of this filtration system is its ability to ionize minerals in water, thereby increasing the mineral bioavailability and the pH. This is an excellent method of eliminating digestive and other problems caused by over-acidity. The machine is ideal because it allows you to adjust the alkaline level of the water you drink, and maintaining an alkaline pH is important for total body health. If you are not completely satisfied with this product, the company will refund your money.

Index

acetyl-l-carnitine, for:
    memory loss, 245;
    stroke, 311
acidophilus (including probiotics), for:
    bruising, 62;
    colon cancer, 74;
    cystitis, 117;
    diverticulitis, 130;
    food poisoning, 152;
    irritable bowel syndrome, 227;
    milk intolerance, 254;
    nosebleeds, 264–65
acne, 1–3
aging spots, 58–61
alcoholics, daily regimen for, 55
allergies, 3–9
aloe vera, for:
    burns, 67
    diverticulosis, 130
    frostbite, 160;
    heartburn and hiatal hernia, 183;
    insect bites, 220;
    ulcers, 320
alpha-lipoic acid, for:
    diabetes, 125;
    hepatitis, 188;
    hypoglycemia, 205
Alzheimer's disease, 9–12
anal itching, 282–85
anemia, 13–16
angelica, for PMS, 279
angina pectoris, 17–19
anorexia nervosa, 19–21
appendicitis, 22–23
arginine, for:

angina pectoris, 18;
    congestive heart failure, 107;
    high blood pressure, 194;
    intermittent claudication, 225
arrhythmias (irregular heartbeats),
    23–25
arthritis, 26–31
asthma, 31–35
astragalus, for:
    arrhythmias, 24;
    bronchitis, 57;
    colds and flu, 104;
    Lyme disease, 239;
    sinusitis, 299
athlete's foot, 156–58
attention deficit disorder/hyper-
    activity (ADD), 35–38
autism, 38–41

back pain, 41–44
bad breath, 44–46
bedsores, 46–48
bedwetting, 49–50
Bell's Palsy, 50–53
benign prostatic hyperplasia, 280
beriberi, 53–55
beta-carotene, for:
    angina pectoris, 18–19;
    cervical and vaginal cancer, 74;
    dizziness, 131
bilberry, for night vision, 243, 262,
    263
bioflavonoids, for:
    bruising, 62;
    bursitis, 69;

bioflavonoids, for: (*cont.*)
  hemorrhoids, 186–87;
  sinusitis, 299;
  stroke, 312
biotin, for dandruff, 120
bladder infections, 116–18
bone softening, 266–68
boron, for:
  back pain, 42;
  osteoporosis, 270
bromelain, for:
  arthritis, 29;
  back pain, 42;
  bursitis, 69;
  gout, 172;
  sinusitis, 299;
  varicose veins, 325
bronchitis, 56–58
brown spots, 58–61
bruising, 61–63
bruxism, 63–64
bulimia, 19–21
bunions, 155
burns, 64–67
bursitis, 68–71

cabbage juice, for ulcers, 321
calcium, for:
  back pain, 42, 43;
  bruxism, 64;
  colon cancer, 74;
  constipation, 109;
  cramps, 111, 112;
  high blood pressure, 193, 194,
    195;
  hyperthyroidism, 202;
  insomnia, 222;
  lead poisoning, 233, 234
  osteomalacia, 267, 268;
  osteoporosis, 270, 271, 272;
  premenstrual syndrome (PMS),
    278, 279;
  restless leg syndrome, 288, 290;
  spina bifida, 303;
  stress, 305
cancer, 71–77
Candida albicans, 77–81
canker sores, 81–83
cardiomyopathy, 83–86
carnitine, for:

cardiomyopathy, 85;
  fatigue, 145
carpal tunnel syndrome, 86–88
cataracts, 88–91
cavities, 91–93
celiac disease, 93–96
cellulite, 96–98
chelation therapy, for:
  Alzheimer's disease, 12;
  angina pectoris, 18;
  autism, 40;
  circulatory disorders, 101;
  impotence, 212;
  intermittent claudication, 226;
  lead poisoning, 234;
  mercury toxicity, 253;
cholesterol levels, 196–98
choline, for Alzheimer's disease,
    10
chondroitin sulphate, for:
  arthritis, 28;
  circulatory disorders, 100
  intermittent claudication, 225
chromium, for:
  diabetes, 125, 126;
  hypoglycemia, 205
chronic fatigue syndrome, 143–48
circulation, poor leg, 224–26
circulatory disorders, 98–102
cluster headaches, 173
Coca Test, for acne, 4, 7
coenzyme Q-10, for:
  arrhythmias, 24, 25;
  breast cancer, 74;
  cardiomyopathy, 84, 85;
  congestive heart failure, 108;
  fatigue, 145;
  gingivitis, 166, 167, 168;
  heart attack, 181;
  high blood pressure, 193, 195;
  infertility/sterility, 217;
  mitral valve prolapse, 258, 259;
  Raynaud's disease, 286
colds and flu, 102–6
congestive heart failure, 106–8
constipation, 108–10; appendicitis
    and, 22
copper, for:
  arthritis, 28;
  cardiomyopathy, 84, 85;

macular degeneration, 242;
osteoporosis, 270;
wrinkles, 334
corns, 155
cramps, 110–13
curcumin, for:
arthritis, 29;
skin cancer, 75
cystic fibrosis, 113–15
cystitis, 116–18

dandelion, for warts, 331, 332
dandruff, 118–20
depression, 121–24
DHEA, for:
Alzheimer's disease, 10–11;
arthritis, 28;
asthma, 33;
bladder cancer, 74
diabetes, 124–26
diarrhea, 127–28
digestion:
acne and poor, 1, 2;
allergies and poor, 8–9;
asthma and, 33–34
diverticulitis, 128–30
dizziness, 131–33
dry eyes, 133–35

ear infections, 135–38
echinacea, for:
canker sores, 82;
colds and flu, 104;
ear infections, 136;
gingivitis, 167;
incontinence, 214;
Lyme disease, 239;
sinusitis, 299
edema, 138–40
emphysema, 140–43
environmental allergens, asthma and, 32, 34
Epstein-Barr virus, 144
evening primrose oil, for:
ADD, 37;
arthritis, 28;
dandruff, 119;
hyperthyroidism, 202;
premenstrual syndrome (PMS), 278, 279;

wrinkles, 333
exercises, for back pain, 43, 44

fatigue, 143–48
fiber, for:
appendicitis, 23;
gallstones, 161;
heartburn and hiatal hernia, 183;
hemorrhoids, 185
fibromyalgia, 148–51
5-HTP, for:
headaches and migraines, 174;
insomnia, 222;
overweight, 273;
stress, 305
flavonoids, for:
bedsores, 47;
ear infections, 136;
hemorrhoids, 185;
scurvy, 294;
ulcers, 320, 321;
varicose veins, 325
flu, 102–6
folic acid, for:
anemia, 14, 15–16;
cancer, 74;
celiac disease, 94, 95;
circulatory disorders, 100, 101;
constipation, 109;
depression, 122, 123;
gout, 171, 172;
intermittent claudication, 225;
osteoporosis, 270;
restless leg syndrome, 289;
for spina bifida, 302–3;
vitiligo, 328–29
folic acid-deficiency anemia, 14
food allergies: 7, 8–9;
arthritis and, 30, 31;
asthma and, 32, 34;
bedwetting and, 49
food poisoning, 151–54
foot problems, 154–58
free radicals, 77, 115
frostbite, 158–60
fungal infections, asthma and, 35

gallstones, 160–62
gamma-linoleic acid (GLA), for:
candida, 79;

gamma-linoleic acid (GLA), for:
(*cont.*)
colds and flu, 104
garlic, for:
arthritis, 29;
asthma, 34;
athlete's foot, 157;
Bell's Palsy, 52;
cancer, 75;
candida, 80;
circulatory disorders, 100;
colds and flu, 104;
cystitis, 117;
diarrhea, 127;
dizziness, 131;
foot problems, 157;
gas, 164;
heart attack, 181;
high blood pressure, 194;
incontinence, 214;
infertility/sterility, 218;
insect bites, 219, 220;
intermittent claudication, 225;
lupus, 236;
Lyme disease, 239;
mercury toxicity, 252;
mitral valve prolapse, 258
gas, 163–65
ginger, for:
arthritis, 29;
dizziness, 131;
food poisoning, 152;
headaches and migraines, 174;
heartburn and hiatal hernia, 183;
motion sickness and morning
sickness, 260;
skin cancer, 75
gingivitis, 165–68
ginkgo biloba, for:
Alzheimer's disease, 11;
asthma, 33;
autism, 40;
dizziness, 131;
dry eyes, 134;
hearing loss, 178;
impotence, 211;
infertility/sterility, 217;
intermittent claudication, 225;
macular degeneration, 242;
memory loss, 245;

Raynaud's disease, 286;
tinnitus, 316, 318
glaucoma, 168–70
glucosamine sulfate, for:
arthritis, 28;
back pain, 42
goldenseal, for:
cystitis, 117;
food poisoning, 152;
gingivitis, 167, 168
sinusitis, 299
gout, 170–73
grapeseed and pine bark extracts, for:
brown spots, 59;
cancer, 75;
stroke, 312
gugglipid, for stroke, 312

halitosis, 44–46
hawthorn, for:
arrhythmias, 25;
cardiomyopathy, 85, 86;
congestive heart failure, 107;
low blood pressure, 195;
lupus, 237
headaches, 173–76
hearing loss, 176–79
heart attack, 179–82
heartburn, 182–84
heel spurs, 155
hemorrhoids, 184–87
hepatitis, 187–89
hernias, 182–84
herpes zoster, 295–98
hiatal hernia, 182–84
hiccups, 190–91
high blood pressure, 192–95
high cholesterol, 196–98
hives, 198–200
homeopathic remedies, for:
arthritis, 30;
constipation, 110;
diarrhea, 127;
diverticulitis, 130;
food poisoning, 154;
frostbite, 160;
insomnia, 223;
menopause, 249;
nosebleeds, 265;
Raynaud's disease, 286;

restless leg syndrome, 289;
   sinusitis, 300
hydrochloric acid, for:
   acne and lack of, 1, 3;
   allergies, 6, 8;
   asthma, 33–34;
   bad breath, 45;
   gas, 164;
   lupus, 236;
   rosacea, 291;
   vitiligo, 328
hyperactivity, 38
hypertension, 192–95
hyperthyroidism, 200–203
hypoglycemia, 203–6
hypothyroidism, 206–10

impotence, 210–13
incontinence, 213–15
infertility/sterility (male), 216–18
inositol, for:
   insomnia, 222;
   intermittent claudication, 225;
   Raynaud's disease, 286
insect bites, 218–20
insomnia, 221–23
intermittent claudication, 224–26
intestinal gas, 163–65
involuntary urination, 213–15
iron, for:
   anemia, 14, 15;
   lead poisoning, 234;
   restless leg syndrome, 289;
   uterine fibroids, 323;
   wrinkles, 334
irregular heartbeats, 23–25
irritable bowel syndrome, 226–28
isoflavones, for menopause, 248

khellin extract, for vitiligo, 328
kidney stones, 229–31

l-arginine, for:
   impotence, 211;
   infertility/sterility, 217
l-carnitine, for:
   angina pectoris, 18;
   arrhythmias, 25;
   cardiomyopathy, 84;
   congestive heart failure, 107;

heart attack, 181;
   infertility/sterility, 217;
   overweight, 273
lactase, for milk intolerance, 254
lactobacillus acidophilus (*See* probiotics), for:
   candida, 80;
   uterine fibroids, 322
lead poisoning, 232–35
lecithin, for:
   gallstones, 161;
   memory loss, 245;
   spina bifida, 302, 303
legs
   poor circulation in, 224–26;
   restless leg syndrome, 288–90
liver spots, 58–61
low blood sugar, 203–6
low thyroid function, 206–10
lupus, 235–38
lycopene, for:
   cancer, 74;
   circulatory disorders, 100;
   emphysema, 142;
   intermittent claudication, 225;
   macular degeneration, 242;
   prostate enlargement, 281
Lyme disease, 238–41

macular degeneration, 241–43
magnesium, for:
   arrhythmias, 24, 25;
   asthma, 34;
   autism, 40, 41;
   back pain, 42;
   bedwetting, 49, 50;
   cardiomyopathy, 84, 85;
   congestive heart failure, 107;
   cramps, 111;
   fatigue, 145, 147;
   fibromyalgia, 149, 150, 151;
   glaucoma, 169;
   headaches and migraines, 174, 175;
   hearing loss, 178, 179;
   heart attack, 181;
   high blood pressure, 193, 195;
   hyperthyroidism, 202, 203;
   hypoglycemia, 206;
   incontinence, 214, 215;
   kidney stones, 230, 231;

magnesium, for: (*cont.*)
  mitral valve prolapse, 258;
  osteomalacia, 267;
  osteoporosis, 270;
  premenstrual syndrome (PMS),
    278;
  Raynaud's disease, 286, 287;
  restless leg syndrome, 289, 290;
  stress, 305, 306–307;
  tinnitus, 317, 318;
  uterine fibroids, 322;
  wrinkles, 333, 334;
malic acid, for fibromylagia, 149, 151;
manganese, for:
  arthritis, 28;
  back pain, 42;
  cystic fibrosis, 114;
  osteoporosis, 270;
  premenstrual syndrome (PMS),
    278;
  tinnitus, 317
melatonin, for:
  fibromyalgia, 149;
  insomnia, 222;
  stress, 305
memory loss, 244–47
menopause, 247–50
mercury toxicity, 251–53
methylsulfonylmethane (MSM), for:
  allergies, 6;
  arthritis, 29
migraines, 173–76
milk tolerance, 253–55
miscarriage, 255–57
mitral valve prolapse, 257–59
morning sickness, 259–61
motion sickness, 259–61
mouthwashes, 46
multivitamin-mineral complex, for:
  anorexia nervosa/bulimia, 20;
  bedwetting, 49;
  beriberi, 54;
  candida, 79;
  cavities, 92;
  cystic fibrosis, 114;
  diverticulitis, 129;
  hyperthyroidism, 201

neuromas, 155
niacin, for:
  arthritis, 29;
  hearing loss, 178
night blindness, 262–63
nosebleeds, 264–66
nux vomica, for:
  insomnia, 223
  sinusitis, 300;

omega-3 essential fatty acids, for:
  circulatory disorders, 100;
  colds and flu, 104;
  dandruff, 119;
  dry eyes, 134;
  high blood pressure, 193;
  lupus, 236, 238;
  prostate enlargement, 281;
  sinusitis, 299
omega-3 oils, for:
  arrhythmias, 24, 25;
  arthritis, 29;
  asthma, 34;
  back pain, 42;
  cancer, 74
osteoarthritis, 26, 27
osteomalacia, 266–68
osteoporosis, 268–72
overweight, 272–75

PC SPES, for prostate cancer, 75
pellagra, 275–77
pernicious anemia, 13, 16
phosphatidylserine, for: memory,
  246, 247
piles, 184–87
poor leg circulation, 224–26
potassium, for:
  cramps, 111, 112;
  high blood pressure, 193, 195;
  premenstrual syndrome, 279;
  restless leg syndrome, 289, 290;
premenstrual syndrome (PMS),
  277–79
primary hypertension, 192–93
probiotics, for:
  bruising, 62;
  colon cancer, 74;
  cystitis, 117;
  diverticulitis, 130;
  food poisoning, 152;
  irritable bowel syndrome, 227;

milk intolerance, 254;
nosebleeds, 264–65
prostate enlargement, 280–82
pruritus ani, 282–85

quercetin, for:
allergies, 6;
asthma, 34;
bursitis, 69;
cancer, 75;
gout, 171;
hives, 199

Raynaud's disease, 285–87
restless leg syndrome, 288–90
rheumatoid arthritis, 26, 27
ringing in the ears, 315–18
Rinkel Rotary Diversified Diet, 4–5
rosacea, 290–93

S-adenosyl, for:
arthritis, 29;
depression, 122
S-adenosylmethionine (SAMe), for
fibromyalgia, 150
St. John's wort, for:
depression, 122;
fibromyalgia, 150;
incontinence, 214
scurvy, 293–95
secondary hypertension, 192
selenium, for:
anemia, 15, 16;
asthma, 34;
Bell's Palsy, 52;
cancer, 75, 77;
cataracts, 89, 90;
cystic fibrosis, 114, 115;
dizziness, 131, 132;
macular degeneration, 242, 243;
mercury toxicity, 252, 253
shark cartilage, for:
arthritis, 29;
cancer, 75
shark liver oil, for:
fatigue, 146;
Lyme disease, 239
shingles, 295–98
sickle cell anemia, 14
sinusitis, 298–301

Sjögren's syndrome, 133–35
sleeplessness, 221–23
spastic colon, 226–28
spina bifida, 301–3
sterility (male), 216–18
stress, 102, 304–7
stretch marks, 307–10
stroke, 310–13
sunburn, 313–15

taurine, for:
arrhythmias, 24;
cardiomyopathy, 84;
congestive heart failure, 107;
edema, 139;
fatigue, 146;
gallstones, 161;
high blood pressure, 193;
macular degeneration, 242
teeth grinding, 63–64
tendonitis, 68
tennis elbow, 68
tension headaches, 173
thyroid hormone, for:
fibromyalgia, 150;
memory loss, 246;
overweight, 274
tinnitus, 315–18
toenail fungus, 156
tryptophan:
depression, 123;
pellagra, 276

ulcers, 319–21
urinary tract infections, 116–18
uterine fibroids, 322–24

varicose veins, 324–27
vertigo, 131–33
vitamin A, for:
acne 1, 2;
allergies, 5, 7;
arthritis, 28;
asthma, 33;
athlete's foot, 156;
bedsores, 47, 48;
Bell's Palsy, 51, 52;
bronchitis, 56, 57;
burns, 66, 67;
bursitis, 69, 70;

vitamin A, for: (*cont.*)
cancer, 73, 76;
cataracts, 89, 90;
colds and flu, 103, 105;
cystic fibrosis, 114, 115;
cystitis, 117–18;
dry eyes, 134;
ear infections, 136;
edema, 139–40;
emphysema, 141, 142;
food poisoning, 152;
gingivitis, 166, 167;
hearing loss, 177, 178;
hemorrhoids, 185;
hypothyroidism, 208, 209;
kidney stones, 230;
Lyme disease, 239;
macular degeneration, 242, 243;
night blindness, 262, 263;
osteomalacia, 267;
osteoporosis, 269;
pruritis ani, 283, 284;
rosacea, 291, 292;
shingles, 296, 297;
sinusitis, 299;
stretch marks, 308, 309;
tinnitus, 316, 317;
ulcers, 320;
varicose veins, 325, 326;
warts, 330, 331;
wrinkles, 333, 334–335;
vitamin B-complex, for:
acne, 1, 2;
allergies, 5, 7;
Alzheimer's disease, 10;
anemia, 15;
anorexia nervosa and bulimia, 20;
arthritis, 28;
asthma, 33;
bad breath, 45;
Bell's Palsy, 51;
beriberi, 54;
bruising, 62;
bruxism, 64;
bursitis, 69;
candida, 79;
canker sores, 82;
cardiomyopathy, 84;
cataracts, 89;
cavities, 92;
celiac disease, 94;
circulatory disorders, 99;
colds and flu, 103;
congestive heart failure, 107;
dandruff, 119;
depression, 122;
diabetes, 125;
diverticulitis, 129;
dry eyes, 134;
edema, 139;'
fatigue, 145;
headaches and migraines, 174;
hearing loss, 177;
heartburn and hiatal hernia, 183;
hyperthyroidism, 201;
hypoglycemia, 205;
hypothyroidism, 208;
impotence, 211;
infertility/sterility, 216;
insect bites, 219;
intermittent claudication, 224;
lead poisoning, 233;
macular degeneration, 242;
memory loss, 245;
osteoporosis, 269;
pellagra, 276;
premenstrual syndrome (PMS), 278;
pruritis ani, 283;
Raynaud's disease, 286;
restless leg syndrome, 288;
spina bifida, 302;
stress, 305;
stretch marks, 308;
tinnitus, 316;
uterine fibroids, 322;
varicose veins, 325;
vitiligo, 328;
wrinkles, 333
vitamin B1, for:
beriberi, 55;
canker sores, 82;
cardiomyopathy, 84, 85;
depression, 122, 123;
memory loss, 246
vitamin B2, for:
headaches and migraines, 174;
hypothyroidism, 209;
rosacea, 291, 292;
stress, 305, 306;

wrinkles, 335
vitamin B3, for memory loss: 245
vitamin B5, for: colds and flu, 103;
  stretch marks, 308
vitamin B6, 316; for:
  anemia, 14, 16;
  asthma, 33;
  autism, 39, 40, 41;
  carpal tunnel syndrome, 87;
  celiac disease, 94, 95;
  circulatory disorders, 99, 101;
  kidney stones, 35;
  motion sickness and morning
    sickness, 260;
  osteoporosis, 270;
  tinnitus, 316, 317;
vitamin B12, for:
  allergies, 5–6;
  Alzheimer's disease, 10, 12;
  anemia, 14–15, 16;
  asthma, 33;
  bursitis, 69, 70–71;
  circulatory disorders, 101;
  dandruff, 119, 120;
  depression, 122, 123;
  fatigue, 145, 147;
  hearing loss, 177;
  hives, 199;
  hypothyroidism, 209;
  infertility/steriligy, 217;
  memory loss, 245, 246;
  osteoporosis, 270;
  shingles, 296;
  spina bifida, 302;
  tinnitus, 316, 318;
  vitiligo, 328;
vitamin C, for:
  acne, 1, 2, 3;
  allergies, 6, 7;
  arthritis, 28;
  asthma, 33;
  athlete's foot, 156;
  back pain, 42;
  bad breath, 45;
  bedsores, 47, 48;
  Bell's Palsy, 51, 52;
  beriberi, 54, 55;

bronchitis, 57;
brown spots, 59, 60;
bruising, 62;
burns, 66, 67;
bursitis, 69, 70;
cancer, 73;
candida, 79;
canker sores, 82–83;
cataracts, 89, 90;
cavities, 92;
cellulite, 97;
circulatory disorders, 100, 101;
colds and flu, 104, 105–6;
constipation, 109;
cystitis, 117, 118;
depression, 122, 123;
diverticulitis, 129;
dizziness, 131, 132;
dry eyes, 134, 135;
ear infections, 136;
edema, 139, 140;
emphysema, 141, 142;
fatigue, 145, 147;
fibromyalgia, 149, 150;
food poisoning, 152;
frostbite, 159;
gallstones, 161;
gingivitis, 166, 167;
glaucoma, 169;
hemorrhoids, 185;
hepatitis, 188;
high blood pressure, 193, 194;
high cholesterol, 197;
hives, 199;
hyperthyroidism, 201, 202;
hypothyroidism, 208, 209;
impotence, 211, 212;
infertility/sterility, 216, 217–218;
intermittent claudication, 224,
  225–226;
kidney stones, 231;
lead poisoning, 233, 234;
lupus, 236, 237;
Lyme disease, 239;
macular degeneration, 242, 243;
mercury toxicity, 252–53;
miscarriage, 256, 257;
nosebleeds, 264;
osteomalacia, 267;

vitamin C, for: *(cont.)*
  osteoporosis, 270;
  pruritis ani, 283, 284;
  rosacea, 291, 292;
  scurvy, 294, 295;
  shingles, 296, 297;
  stress, 305, 306;
  stretch marks, 308, 309;
  stroke, 311, 312;
  sunburn, 314;
  ulcers, 320, 321;
  varicose veins, 325, 326;
  vitiligo, 328, 329;
  warts, 330. 331;
  wrinkles, 333, 33
vitamin D, f
  back pain, 42;
  celiac disease, 94, 95;
  cramps, 111, 112;
  cystic fibrosis, 114, 115;
  hearing loss, 178;
  hyperthyroidism, 201, 203;
  osteomalacia, 267;
  osteoporosis, 270, 272;
  stress, 305, 306;
vitamin E, for:
  acne, 2, 3;
  Alzheimer's disease, 10, 12;
  anemia, 15, 16;
  arthritis, 28;
  asthma, 33;
  Bell's Palsy, 52;
  beriberi, 54, 55;
  bronchitis, 57, 58;
  brown spots, 59, 60;
  burns, 66, 67;
  cancer, 74, 76–77;
  cataracts, 89, 90;
  circulatory disorders, 100, 101;
  cramps, 111;
  cystic fibrosis, 114;
  dandruff, 119, 120;
  edema, 139, 140;
  emphysema, 142;
  fatigue, 145, 147;
  gingivitis, 166, 167;
  gout, 171, 172;
  heart attack, 181;
  hepatitis, 188;
  hyperthyroidism, 201, 202–203;

  hypothyroidism, 208, 209;
  infertility/sterility, 217, 218;
  intermittent claudication, 225, 226;
  lead poisoning, 233, 234;
  lupus, 236, 237;
  macular degeneration, 243;
  menopause, 248;
  miscarriage, 256;
  premenstrual syndrome (PMS), 288, 289, 278;
  prostate en..., 288, 289,
  Ray...,
  shingles, 296, 297;
  spina bifida, 302, 303;
  stretch marks, 309;
  sunburn, 314;
  varicose veins, 325, 326;
  warts, 330, 331;
  wrinkles, 333, 334;
vitamin K, for osteoporosis, 270
vitiligo, 327–29

warts, 329–32
water, for:
  acne and, 1, 2;
  allergies and, 7;
  Alzheimer's disease and
      aluminum levels in water,
      11, 12;
  appendicitis and, 22;
  bedsores and, 47;
  bronchitis and, 57;
  brown spots and, 60;
  burns and, 67;
  bursitis and, 70;
  cancer and, 76;
  candida and, 80;
  cataracts and, 90;
  cellulite and, 97;
  circulatory disorders and, 101;
  colds and flu and, 105;
  constipation and, 109;
  cramps and, 112;
  cystitis and, 117;
  diarrhea and, 128;
  diverticulitis and, 130;
  fatigue and, 147;
  fibromyalgia and, 150;

food poisoning and, 153;
gallstones and, 162;
gingivitis and, 167;
gout and, 172;
heart attack and, 181;
heartburn and hiatal hernia and, 184;
hemorrhoids and, 186;
high blood pressure and, 194;
high cholesterol and, 197;
hypothyroidism and, 209;
incontenince and, 215;
irritable bowel syndrome and, 228;
kidney stones and, 230;
menopause and, 249;
mercury toxicity and, 252;
overweight and, 273;
premenstrual syndrome (PMS) and, 278;
rosacea and, 292;
shingles and, 297;
sinusitis and, 300;
stretch marks and, 309;
sunburn and, 314;
varicose veins and, 326;
wrinkles and, 334
water retention, 138–40
white spots or patches, 327–29
wrinkles, 332–35

yeast overgrowth, 77–81

zinc, for:
    acne 2, 3;
    Alzheimer's disease, 11, 12;
    anemia, 15, 16;
    anorexia nervosa and bulimia, 20, 21;
    arthritis, 29;
    athlete's foot, 156;
    bedsores, 47, 48;
    Bell's Palsy, 52;
    bronchitis, 57, 58;
    burns, 66, 67;
    bursitis, 69, 70;
    cancer, 75;
    cardiomyopathy, 85;
    colds and flu, 104, 105;
    cystitis, 117, 118;
    diabetes, 125, 126;
    ear infections, 136;
    food poisoning, 152;
    gingivitis, 167;
    hemorrhoids, 185–86;
    high blood pressure, 194, 195;
    impotence, 211, 212;
    infertility/sterility, 217, 218;
    kidney stones, 230;
    lead poisoning, 233, 234;
    lupus, 236, 237;
    Lyme disease, 239;
    macular degeneration, 242, 243;
    night blindness, 262, 263;
    prostate enlargement, 281, 282;
    pruritus ani, 283, 284;
    rosacea, 292;
    shingles, 296, 297;
    sinusitis, 299;
    stress, 305, 307;
    stretch marks, 309;
    tinnitus, 317, 318;
    ulcers, 320, 321;
    varicose veins, 325, 326

About Stephen Langer, M.D.

Over the years, Stephen Langer, M.D., has written many health and nutrition articles and columns for numerous publications, among them, *Alternative Medicine, Science Digest,* and *Let's Live* magazine. He has authored three books with James F. Scheer: *Raise Your I.Q., How to Win at Weight Loss,* and *Solved: The Riddle of Illness.* The latter was characterized by Dr. Wayne Dyer as "one of the most important books of our time." Dr. Langer and James Scheer have written more than 20 health booklets.

Dr. Langer has hosted health and nutrition radio and television interview shows in the San Francisco area for many years. General Nutrition Corporation (GNC) sponsored his *Medicine Man* interview show on the Family Channel for more than two years. His latest television interview show, *Feeling Great,* is now in production.

Dr. Langer has been a guest on many national television and radio programs, including *The Oprah Winfrey Show.* He is well known for having made a nationwide tour of major radio and television stations to introduce and popularize evening primrose oil.

Dr. Langer has been a featured speaker on thyroid function at the annual American Academy of Anti-Aging Medicine seminar in Las Vegas and at various nutrition and health conferences in England, Belgium, and France.

Dr. Langer practices Preventative Medicine and Clinical Nutrition at Berkeley, California, where he also resides. He specializes in the treatment of chronic fatigue, fibromyalgia, hypothyroidism thyroiditis, food allergies, and other conditions. He can be reached for personal consultation at 510-548-7384 or 3031 Telegraph Avenue, Suite 230, Berkeley, California 94705.

About James F. Scheer

James F. Scheer is the past editor of three nutrition health publications: *Let's Live, Food-Wise,* and *Health Freedom News.* He now devotes all his time to writing books.

Most of his 22 published books are in the health and nutrition field. The best known are *Foods That Heal,* written with Maureen Salaman; *Solved: The Riddle of Illness,* with Dr. Stephen Langer; and *Raise Your I.Q.,* also with Dr. Langer.

More than 2,000 of James Scheer's articles and columns have appeared in over 100 publications, among them, *Cosmopolitan, Good Housekeeping, Redbook, Esquire, Better Homes and Gardens,* and *Let's Live* magazine.

James Scheer has made hundreds of public appearances and has appeared on countless radio and television shows. While editor of *Let's Live,* he was invited to be a guest on the daily nationally syndicated program *Health Club of the Air.* Because he elicited such an enthusiastic response from his first appearance, he was invited to be a regular guest 2 to 3 times weekly for more than 2½ years.

One of James Scheer's books in a field other than health was used as the basis for Hollywood producer David Wolper's 60-minute documentary *The Race for Space,* a nominee for an Academy Award and winner in its category at the San Francisco International Film Festival.

James Scheer lives in Rancho Mirage, California.

New Perspectives in Health Care
from Kensington Books